EMERGENCY CARDIOLOGY

EMERGENCY CARDIOLOGY

AN EVIDENCE-BASED GUIDE TO ACUTE CARDIAC PROBLEMS

Second Edition

Karim Ratib MBChB BSc(Hons) MRCP
Specialist Registrar in Cardiology, University Hospital of North
Staffordshire, Stoke-on-Trent, UK

Gurbir Bhatia MBChB MD MRCP
Specialist Registrar in Cardiology, University Hospital of North
Staffordshire, Stoke-on-Trent, UK

Neal Uren MD (Hons) FRCP
Consultant Cardiologist, Edinburgh Heart Centre, Royal Infirmary,
Edinburgh, UK

James Nolan MBChB MD FRCP
Consultant Cardiologist, University Hospital of North Staffordshire,
Stoke-on-Trent, UK

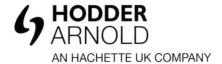

HODDER
ARNOLD
AN HACHETTE UK COMPANY

First published in Great Britain in 2003 by Hodder Arnold
This second edition published in 2010 by
Hodder Education, an Hachette UK Company,
338 Euston Road, London NW1 3BH

http://www.hodderarnold.com

Whilst the advice and information in this book are believed to be true and accurate at the
date of going to press, neither the author[s] nor the publisher can accept any legal
responsibility or liability for any errors or omissions that may be made. In particular (but
without limiting the generality of the preceding disclaimer) every effort has been made to
check drug dosages; however it is still possible that errors have been missed. Furthermore,
dosage schedules are constantly being revised and new side-effects recognized. For these
reasons the reader is strongly urged to consult the drug companies' printed instructions
before administering any of the drugs recommended in this book.

British Library Cataloguing in Publication Data
A catalogue record for this book is available from the British Library

Library of Congress Cataloging-in-Publication Data
A catalog record for this book is available from the Library of Congress

ISBN-13   978 0 340 974 223
1 2 3 4 5 6 7 8 9 10

Commissioning Editor:	Caroline Makepeace
Project Editor:	Sarah Penny
Production Controller:	Kate Harris
Cover Designer:	Lynda King
Indexer:	David Bennett

Typeset in Minion Pro 9.5pt by MPS Limited, A Macmillan Company
Printed and bound in India by Replika Press Pvt Ltd

What do you think about this book? Or any other Hodder Arnold title?
Please visit our website: www.hodderarnold.com

CONTENTS

ABBREVIATIONS

ACC	American College of Cardiology
ACD	active and compression–decompression
ACE	angiotensin converting enzyme
ACS	acute coronary syndrome
ACT	activated clotting time
ADP	adenosine diphosphate
AF	atrial fibrillation
AHA	American Heart Association
aPTT	activated partial thromboplastin time
ATP	adenosine triphosphate
A-V	arteriovenous
AV	atrioventricular
AVNRT	atrioventricular nodal re-entry tachycardia
AVRT	atrioventricular re-entry tachycardia
BP	blood pressure
BSAC	British Society of Antimicrobial Chemotherapy
CABG	coronary artery bypass graft
CAD	coronary artery disease
cAMP	cyclic adenosine monophosphate
CCS	Canadian Cardiovascular Society
CCU	coronary care unit
CK	creatine kinase
CMV	cytomegalovirus
COPD	chronic obstructive pulmonary disease
CPR	cardiopulmonary resuscitation
CRP	C-reactive protein
CT	computed tomography
CTPA	computed tomography pulmonary angiography
CVA	cerebrovascular accident
DAPT	dual antiplatelet therapy
DCC	direct current cardioversion
DES	drug-eluting stent
DVT	deep venous thrombosis
ECG	electrocardiogram
EF	ejection fraction

ELISA	enzyme-linked immunoadsorbent assay
EMD	electromechanical dissociation
EPS	electrophysiological study
ERC	European Resuscitation Council
ESR	erythrocyte sedimentation rate
ESC	European Society of Cardiology
FDP	fibrin degradation products
GI	gastrointestinal
GP	glycoprotein
GRF	gelatin–resorcinol–formaldehyde
GTN	glyceryl trinitrate
HIT	heparin-induced thrombocytopenia
IABP	intra-aortic balloon counterpulsation
IAC	interposed abdominal compression
ICD	implantable cardioverter defibrillator
IE	infective endocarditis
IHD	ischaemic heart disease
IMH	intramural haematoma
INR	international normalized ratio
IPG	impedance plethysmography
IRA	infarct-related artery
IRAD	International Registry of Acute Aortic Dissection
IV	intravenous
IVDU	intravenous druge user
JVP	jugular venous pressure
LAD	left anterior descending (artery)
LIMA	left internal mammary artery
LMWH	low molecular weight heparin
LSD	lysergic acid diethylamide
LVF	left ventricular failure
MACE	major adverse cardiac event
MEN	multiple endocrine neoplasia
MI	myocardial infarction
MIC	minimum inhibitory concentration
MRI	magnetic resonance imaging
MRSA	methecillin resitant staphyloccocus aureus
NICE	National Institute for Health and Clinical Excellence
NPCT	non-penetrating cardiac trauma
NSTEACS	non-ST elevation ACS
NSTEMI	non-ST elevation MI
PAU	penetrating atherosclerotic ulceration

PCI	percutaneous coronary intervention
PE	pulmonary embolism
PEA	pulseless electrical activity
PLS	posterior leucoencephalopathy syndrome
po	per os (orally)
PTCA	percutaneous transluminal coronary angioplasty
PTD	percutaneous thrombolytic device
PTFE	polytetrafluoroethylene
SBP	systolic blood pressure
SC	subcutaenous
SLE	systemic lupus erythematosus
STEMI	ST elevation MI
SVT	supraventricular tachycardia
TCAD	tricyclic antidepressant
TIA	transient ischaemic attack
TOE	transoesophageal echocardiogram (echocardiography)
tPA	tissue plasminogen activator
TVR	target vessel revascularization
UA	unstable angina
UFH	unfractionated heparin
V/Q	ventilation/perfusion
VF	ventricular fibrillation
VT	ventricular tachycardia
WCC	white cell count
WPW	Wolff–Parkinson–White (syndrome)

ACUTE CORONARY SYNDROMES

EPIDEMIOLOGY

Coronary heart disease is the most common cause of death in the United Kingdom. In total, 220 000 deaths were attributable to ischaemic heart disease in 2007. It is estimated that the incidence of acute coronary syndrome (ACS) is over 250 000 per year.

Sudden death remains a frequent complication of ACS: approximately 50 per cent of patients with ST elevation myocardial infarction (STEMI) do not survive, with around two-thirds of the deaths occurring shortly after the onset of symptoms and before admission to hospital. Prior to the development of modern drug regimes and reperfusion strategies, hospital mortality after admission with ACS was 30–40 per cent. After the introduction of coronary care units in the 1960s, outcome was improved, predominantly reflecting better treatment of arrhythmias. Current therapy has improved outcome further for younger patients who present early in the course of their ACS. The last decade has seen a significant fall in the overall 30-day mortality rate. Most patients who die before discharge do so in the first 48 hours after admission, usually due to cardiogenic shock consequent upon extensive left ventricular damage. Most patients who survive to hospital discharge do well, with 90 per cent surviving at least 1 year. Surviving patients who are at increased risk of early death can be identified by a series of adverse clinical and investigational features, and their prognosis improved by intervention.

DEFINITIONS

The term 'acute coronary syndrome' (ACS) has been developed to describe the collection of ischaemic conditions that include a spectrum of diagnoses from unstable angina (UA) to non-ST elevation MI (NSTEMI) and STEMI. Patients presenting with ACS can be classified into two groups according to their electrocardiogram (ECG) (Figure 1.1): those with persistent STEMI and those without (non-ST elevation ACS or NSTEACS). The treatment of STEMI requires emergency restoration of blood flow within an occluded culprit coronary artery. Patients presenting with NSTEACS often have ECG changes including T-wave inversion, ST depression or transient ST elevation, although occasionally the ECG may be entirely normal. This group can be classified further according to the presence of detectable levels of cardiac proteins, troponins, in patients' serum (see below). Thus, NSTEACS patients with undetectable cardiac troponins (UA) are distinguished from those in whom myocardial ischaemia is severe enough to cause myocardial necrosis, leading to troponin release into the circulation (NSTEMI). Detection of cardiac troponin following ACS is a strong predictor of recurrent ischaemia. However, it should be remembered that patients with UA are still at increased risk of further events, especially those with pain at rest or dynamic ST changes on their ECG.

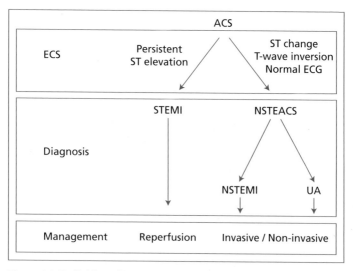

Figure 1.1 Definition, diagnosis and management of ACS.

Myocardial infarction can also be classified with regards to underlying aetiology as defined by the European Society of Cardiology:

Type 1 Spontaneous myocardial infarction related to ischaemia due to a primary coronary event such as plaque erosion and/or rupture, fissuring or dissection.

Type 2 Myocardial infarction secondary to ischaemia due to either increased oxygen demand or decreased supply, e.g. coronary artery spasm, coronary embolism, anaemia, arrhythmias, hypertension or hypotension.

Type 3 Sudden unexpected cardiac death, including cardiac arrest, often with symptoms suggestive of myocardial ischaemia, accompanied by presumably new ST elevation, or new LBBB, or evidence of fresh thrombus in a coronary artery by angiography and/or at autopsy, but death occurring before blood samples could be obtained, or at a time before the appearance of cardiac biomarkers in the blood.

Type 4a Myocardial infarction associated with PCI (percutaneous coronary intrervention).

Type 4b Myocardial infarction associated with stent thrombosis as documented by angiography or at autopsy.

Type 5 Myocardial infarction associated with CABG (coronary artery bypass graft).

PATHOPHYSIOLOGY

ACSs are caused by an imbalance between myocardial oxygen demand and supply that results in cell death and myocardial necrosis. Primarily, this occurs due to factors affecting the coronary arteries, but may also occur as a result of secondary processes such as hypoxaemia or hypotension and factors that increase myocardial oxygen demand. The commonest cause is rupture or erosion of an atherosclerotic plaque that leads to complete occlusion of the artery or partial occlusion with distal embolization of thrombotic material.

Atherosclerosis is a disease of large and medium-sized arteries, affecting predominantly the arterial intima. The precise mechanism responsible for the generation of atherosclerotic arterial disease remains open to debate, but it is likely that arterial endothelial injury is an initiating factor. It is clear that the extent and stability of atherosclerotic lesions is influenced by the common risk factors of smoking, hypertension, hyperlipidaemia and diabetes. There are a large number of other modifiable risk factors, such as homocysteine, oxidative stress, fibrinogen and psychosocial factors, which may play an important role in atherogenesis in some individuals. Individual susceptibility to the adverse effects of risk factors may relate to genetic predisposition.

Atherosclerotic plaques are complex structures consisting of a fibrous cap and a core of lipid, connective tissue and inflammatory cells. The morphology of plaques is variable, and those with a thin fibrous cap, a large lipid core and an increase in inflammatory activity are highly unstable. An increase in inflammatory activity within plaques may be triggered by systemic infections (*Chlamydia*, cytomegalovirus (CMV), *Helicobacter* or chronic dental sepsis) or stimuli such as stress, severe exercise and temperature change. ACS is initiated when the fibrous cap of an unstable atherosclerotic lesion ruptures (in 75 per cent of cases) or the overlying endothelium erodes (in 25 per cent of cases). Plaque erosion is more common in females. Both mechanisms expose highly thrombogenic subendothelial and core components of the unstable plaque to the blood, leading to localized platelet adhesion, activation of the clotting mechanism, and formation of an intraluminal thrombus that occludes the coronary artery. Prior to plaque rupture or erosion, other conformational changes may occur as a result of endothelial injury. This causes a proliferation of smooth muscle cells leading to a reduction of the luminal diameter, which increases shear stress, and causes further endothelial injury. Intravascular ultrasound studies have confirmed that unstable coronary plaques are associated with more expansive arterial remodelling compared to stable coronary lesions, which may imply a more marked recent progression in extent and severity of plaque at the site of rupture/erosion. Angiographic and intravascular ultrasound studies of culprit lesions have demonstrated complex eccentric morphology consistent with ruptured plaque and superimposed thrombus. Vulnerable plaques that fissure or rupture are characterized by large eccentric lipid pools with foam cell infiltration and tend to rupture at the border of the fibrous cap and adjacent normal intima. This weakness in the integrity of the plaque is initiated by matrix metalloproteinases secreted by macrophages, and ultimately rupture occurs through an acute change in wall shear stress.

The lipid core is a potent substrate for platelet-rich thrombus formation with the initiation of the coagulation cascade through the interaction of tissue factor with factor VIIa. Platelet adhesion to subendothelial collagen through the release of tissue factor and the expression of the vitronectin ($\alpha_v \beta_3$) receptors leading to platelet activation and aggregation through the expression of the glycoprotein IIb/IIIa receptor is an important event in the development of thrombus. Platelet-rich thrombus is associated with cyclical reductions in coronary blood flow with additional coronary vasoconstriction resulting from endothelial disruption, and thromboxane A_2 (TXA_2) and serotonin production leading to reduced nitric oxide (NO) production. Inflammatory acute phase proteins, cytokines and systemic catecholamines stimulate the production of tissue factor, procoagulant activity and platelet hypercoagulability.

A number of factors that can trigger the onset of ACS have been identified, acting by initiating plaque rupture or promoting thrombus formation. Some patients report heavy physical exertion or mental stress shortly before the onset of ACS. Circadian variation in coagulation and autonomic nervous system activity contribute to an increased incidence of ACS in the morning. Irrespective of this, the risk of an individual episode of exercise or stress precipitating the onset of ACS is low, and most episodes have no identifiable direct triggers.

Other non-athersclerotic causes for ACS include arteritis, trauma, spontaneous coronary dissection, thromboembolism, cocaine use and congenital abnormalities such as anomalous coronary arteries. Patients who present as a result of these rare causes will usually not have the classical risk factors associated with atherosclerosis; typically the diagnosis is not established until after coronary angiography.

Acute STEMI usually results from total occlusion of a coronary artery, with subsequent myocardial cell necrosis occurring in as little as 15 minutes. Continued occlusion results in a wavefront of necrosis spreading from the subendocardium to the subepicardium. The amount of myocardial injury depends on the duration of occlusion, the presence of collateral blood flow and the degree of preconditioning of the myocytes to ischaemia. In animal models, persistent occlusion of a coronary artery will usually result in complete infarction of the area subtended after 6 hours. Subendocardial and full thickness or transmural mycocardial infarction can be well demonstrated with cardiac magnetic resonance imaging (MRI) using late gadolinium enhanced images. These images correlate well with macroscopic histological findings.

NSTEACS are usually associated with partial or transient occlusion of the coronary artery that may result in ST depression or T-wave changes on the ECG. Myocardial injury occurs as a result of a sudden decrease in luminal diameter leading to reduced perfusion or due to plaque rupture/erosion and embolization of thrombotic material into the distal coronary bed. Most individuals with atherosclerotic coronary artery disease have a large number of minor lesions that do not significantly narrow the coronary lumen, as well as a smaller number of severe lesions. The severe lesions are more likely to intermittently limit antegrade blood flow during exercise (leading to stable angina). An ACS is more likely to occur due to instability in one of the more numerous minor lesions (two-thirds of ACS are related to angiographically minor lesions). Intravascular ultrasound studies have shown that patients with NSTEACS frequently have multiple ruptured plaques often occurring in arteries other than the initial culprit.

UA can be caused by the same mechanisms as NSTEMI, although the detectable myocardial necrosis does not usually occur. UA may also be caused by a reduction in coronary flow due to a decrease in luminal diameter caused by increase in size of a non-ruptured plaque where endothelial damage leads to smooth muscle proliferation. For these reasons, patients even with negative biomarkers may still be at high risk of further events and this reinforces the need for effective risk stratification.

DIAGNOSIS

Presentation

Chest pain is a common reason for patients to attend hospital, accounting for up to 5 per cent of visits to the emergency department and 40 per cent of hospital admissions. Around 50 per cent of patients presenting with chest pain will have an underlying ACS, requiring hospitalization and intensive medical therapy. The remainder have other cardiac and non-cardiac causes for their symptoms, and require a different management approach. This section gives guidelines on diagnosing ACS, and differentiating it from other common causes of chest pain.

The diagnosis of ACS is usually made using a combination of clinical and ECG features. Cardiac troponin studies and functional tests can then be used to further risk-stratify the patient. As a general principle, all patients with symptoms that may be due to an ACS should be admitted to hospital. These patients should preferably be admitted to a chest pain assessment unit or heart attack centre, as those at high risk of early adverse events need to be carefully monitored and selected for early invasive therapy.

Clinical features

Most patients with ACS present with chest discomfort; in STEMI and 80 per cent of NSTEACS this is prolonged, lasting over 20 minutes.

Accelerated or recent onset angina is present in 20 per cent of patients with NSTEACS, where the pain is intermittent and related to stress or exertion. Typically, the discomfort is retrosternal, crushing and severe, radiating to the neck, arms or back. There is often associated nausea, sweating and vomiting related to the release of toxins from injured myocardial cells and autonomic activation. It is not usually affected by changes in posture, movement or respiration. The pain can be atypical (sited in the epigastrium, neck, arms or back or unusual in character). Particularly with inferior infarction, the pain can be difficult to distinguish from dyspepsia. Atypical symptoms are more likely to be present in the young (age 25–40), elderly patients (age > 75), females, those with diabetes, chronic renal failure and those with dementia. In some patients, the pain is minimal or absent, with the dominant symptoms consisting of nausea, vomiting, dyspnoea, weakness, dizziness or syncope (or a combination of these). Occasionally ACS is recognized coincidentally (and often retrospectively) by the presence of ECG abnormalities in addition to raised biochemical markers. It is also important to differentiate those with non-cardiac chest pain from those with anginal symptoms. Typical angina is defined by the presence of all three of the features listed:

- a constricting discomfort across the chest and/or neck, shoulders, jaw or arms
- being precipitated by physical exertion or psychological stress
- relieved by rest or by nitrogycerin within about 5 minutes.

If only two of the above features are present, it is considered to be atypical angina. If one or none of these features are present, the patient is considered to have non-anginal chest pain. Angina is less likely if the pain is unrelated to activity, brought on by inspiration, or associated with syptoms such as palpitations, tingling or dysphagia. If non-anginal chest pain is diagnosed, another cause for the pain shoud be considered.

Electrocardiographic changes

The majority of patients with an ACS will have an abnormal ECG at some stage. An initial normal ECG does not rule out the diagnosis, as ECG changes can develop, evolve and resolve rapidly. Commonly, the first ECG performed during the course of the presentation (often by paramedics) is the one that shows evidence of myocardial ischaemia, prior to resolution with appropriate pre-hospital treatment. Patients with a suggestive history and a normal ECG should be admitted and the ECG monitored at regular intervals; if ECG changes then develop, appropriate treatment can be initiated.

STEMI is diagnosed by the presence of characteristic chest pain for more than 30 minutes and ST-segment elevation of ≥ 2 mV (2 mm) in two or more contiguous precordial leads or ≥ 1 mV (1 mm) in two or more adjacent limb leads or new left bundle branch block. In patients with this type of evolving MI:

- ST elevation develops rapidly (30–60 seconds) after coronary occlusion, and is usually associated with prolonged total occlusion of a coronary artery.

- The ST elevation resolves over several hours in response to spontaneous or therapeutic coronary reperfusion. Persistent ST elevation is a sign of failure to reperfuse, and is associated with a large infarct and an adverse prognosis. T-wave inversion, pathological Q waves and loss of R waves often develop in the infarct zone when reperfusion has been late or incomplete, indicating the presence of extensive myocardial necrosis. When successful reperfusion occurs early in the course of an evolving ST elevation MI, there may be little myocardial necrosis, preservation of the R waves and no Q-wave formation. Occasionally, reperfusion therapy may be administered so rapidly that any infarction is aborted.

In a small proportion of patients with chest pain and evolving MI (around 5 per cent) the presenting ECG demonstrates bundle branch block (usually left). This is commonly associated with extensive anterior infarction and a poor prognosis. The distribution of ECG changes provides some information on the area of myocardium involved:

- Changes in V2–V6 indicate anterior ischaemia or necrosis in the territory of the left anterior descending (LAD) artery. Extensive infarction in this territory is associated with a high risk of heart failure, arrhythmias, mechanical complications and early death (Figure 1.2).

- Changes in I, aVL, V5 and V6 indicate lateral ischaemia or necrosis in the territory of the circumflex artery or diagonal branches of the LAD (Figure 1.3). Infarction in this territory has a better prognosis than extensive anterior infarction.

- Changes in II, III and a VF indicate inferior ischaemia or necrosis in the territory of the right coronary artery (Figure 1.4, page 12). Compared with patients with extensive anterior infarction, these patients have a lower incidence of heart failure, an increased incidence of bradyarrhythmias (since atrioventricular (AV) nodal ischaemia or vagal activation often accompanies occlusion of the right coronary artery) and a relatively good prognosis.

- Tall R waves in V1–V3 associated with ST depression indicate ischaemia or necrosis in the posterior wall, often associated with circumflex or right coronary artery occlusion (Figure 1.5, page 13).

NSTEACS are associated with transient ST segment changes (≥ 0.5 mm) that develop with symptoms at rest and which may resolve with the resolution of symptoms. The degree of ST change correlates with the risk of further events and death; those with ≥ 1 mm of ST depression have an 11 per cent risk of MI and death at 1 year whereas those with ≥ 2 mm have 14 per cent risk at 1 year. Transient ST elevation is also associated with a poorer outcome. T-wave inversion and ST changes of < 0.5 mm are less specific at indicating and predicting events, though deep T-wave inversion in leads V2–V6 is associated with disease in the proximal LAD. Older patients with widespread severe ST depression often have multivessel disease and a poor prognosis. In one study of 773 patients presenting consecutively to hospital within 12 hours of chest pain (without ST segment elevation), 20 per cent had ST-segment depression, 26 per cent had inverted T waves, 11 per cent had a non-diagnostic ECG (bundle branch block, paced rhythm) and 43 per cent had a normal initial ECG. Those patients with normal and minor changes on ECG often have ischaemia in the circumflex territory that may be better detected with use of posterior and right-sided leads.

Diagnostic biochemical markers

Cardiac enzyme studies are employed to substantiate or refute a provisional diagnosis of NSTEMI or UA, and guide further therapy. Myocardial necrosis results in the release of intracellular proteins, which can be detected in blood samples. Measurement of total creatine kinase (CK) level has been employed as a common biochemical test in patients with suspected MI, with a temporally related increase to more than twice the upper limit of normal regarded as diagnostic. CK is widely distributed in non-cardiac tissues, and therefore has a significant rate of false-positive results. The isoenzyme, CK-MB, is predominantly located in the myocardium, and for this reason was previously the gold standard marker for myocardial necrosis. A low-molecular-weight protein, myoglobin, is released as a result of damage to any muscle. Whilst non-specific for myocardial injury, myoglobin release occurs relatively soon after MI,

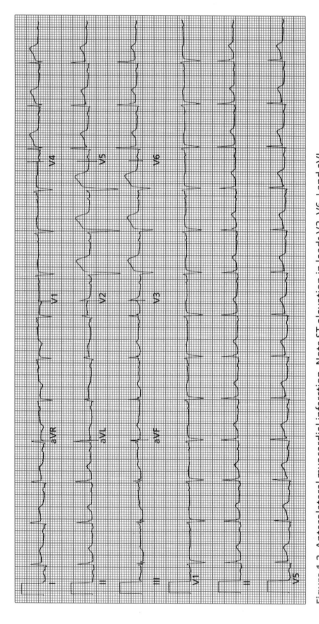

Figure 1.2 Anterolateral myocardial infarction. Note ST elevation in leads V2–V6, I and aVL.

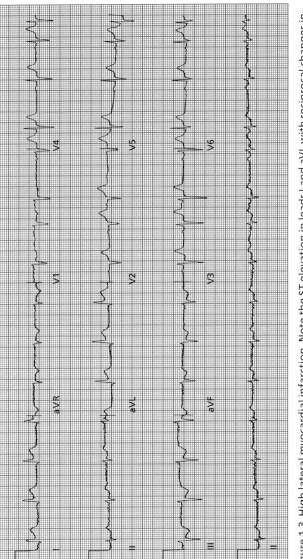

Figure 1.3 High lateral myocardial infarction. Note the ST elevation in leads I and aVL with reciprocal changes in the inferior leads. Coronary angiography demonstrated a 95 per cent stenosis in a high diagonal branch.

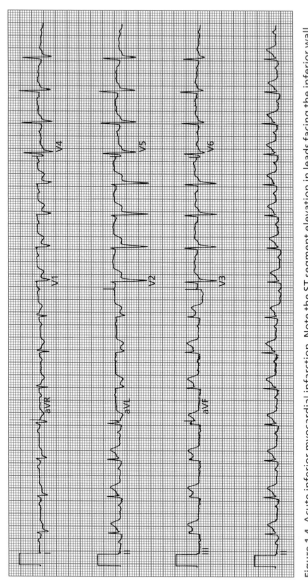

Figure 1.4 Acute inferior myocardial infarction. Note the ST segment elevation in leads facing the inferior wall (II, III, aVF). Reciprocal changes are seen in diametrically opposed leads (I and aVL) located in the same (frontal) plane.

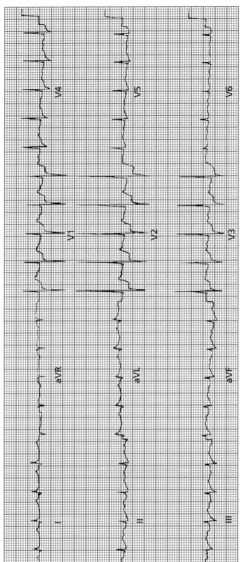

Figure 1.5 Posterior wall myocardial infarction. Note the tall R waves in leads V1–V3 associated with ST depression.

and levels can be detectable within 2 hours, making it a useful early biomarker in the triage of patients with chest pain in the emergency department.

Within the last decade, cardiac troponins have superseded other biomarkers in the detection of myocardial necrosis by virtue of their sensitivity and specificity. Any patient who demonstrates a typical rise and gradual fall of troponin in association with ischaemic symptoms or ECG changes should be diagnosed as having had a definite MI. The troponin complex is an integral part of the cardiac myofibril and is released following damage to myocardium. Two regulatory components, troponin I and T, released by myocardial micro-infarction, can be detected peripherally, indicating that myocardial necrosis has occurred. As well as their specificity, cardiac troponins are highly sensitive, with detectable elevations occurring after necrosis of less than 1 g of myocardial tissue. Troponins are detectable 3–4 hours after the onset of infarction, peak at 12 hours, and can remain elevated for up to 2 weeks. False-positive results can be due to:

- renal failure
- pulmonary embolism
- septicaemia
- rhabdomyolysis
- acute neurological disease (stroke or subarachnoid haemorrhage)
- significant valvular disease (aortic stenosis)
- acute and chronic heart failure
- cardiomyopathy (hypertrophic, apical ballooning)
- infiltrative disease (amyloidosis, sarcoid, haemochromatosis, scleroderma)
- inflammatory disease (myocarditis or myocardial extension of pericarditis and endocarditis)
- cardiotoxic drugs (anthracyclines, herceptin and 5-fluorouracil)
- cardiac contusion
- tachycardia or bradycardia.

Other causes of chest pain

Non-cardiac chest pain can arise from:

- The aorta in acute dissection. The pain of aortic dissection is severe and of sudden onset; it is tearing in nature, often radiates to the back, and may be associated with hypertension, aortic regurgitation, neurological signs and pulse deficits (see Chapter 5).

- The pleura in pneumonia, pulmonary embolism (PE) or pneumothorax. Pain arising from the pleura is unilateral, sharp and stabbing, and worse on inspiration. There may be associated signs of pneumonia, PE or deep venous thrombosis. The majority of patients with pulmonary embolus have no ECG changes apart from a tachycardia or atrial fibrillation (AF). The 'classic' ECG changes of $S_1Q_3T_3$ or right heart strain are associated with large PE and are often transient and easily missed. In spontaneous pneumothorax, there may be central chest pain with few auscultatory signs. Spontaneous pneumothorax is a strong possibility in patients with chronic obstructive pulmonary disease (COPD) who present with chest pain and dyspnoea in the absence of ECG evidence of acute myocardial ischaemia. A chest x-ray is vital to rule out the presence of air in the pleural space.

- The upper gastrointestinal (GI) tract in oesophageal reflux, peptic ulcer disease or cholelithiasis. Dyspeptic pain arising from the upper GI tract is usually burning in nature, may have a clear relationship to posture or food, and is often relieved by antacids. Oesophageal pain may, however, be very similar to the pain of cardiac ischaemia. Exercise-induced oesophageal pain mimicking angina has been well described. In some individuals, oesophageal spasm may occur in association with ST segment change. Nitrates and calcium antagonists will relieve the pain of oesophageal spasm. Correct diagnosis in these difficult patients requires coronary arteriography, investigations to rule out coronary spasm, myocardial perfusion imaging and ambulatory oesophageal pH and pressure monitoring.

- The pericardium in pericarditis. Pericardial pain is retrosternal, sharp, eased by sitting forward, and may worsen with inspiration. It is commonly seen following MI, or in a young adult with acute post-viral pericarditis. A pericardial rub is common, although it may be intermittent. Diagnostic widespread concave ST elevation may be present.

- The bones and muscles in musculoskeletal disorders. Musculoskeletal chest pain is usually unilateral, localized and sharp. It is exacerbated by movement or local pressure. There may be a history of trauma.

- The skin in acute dermatological conditions. Acute skin conditions can (rarely) produce chest pain. The unilateral pain of shingles precedes the rash, and may confuse the unwary.

- Outside the chest cavity. For example, referred pain from the neck. Pain referred from the cervical or thoracic spine will have features of musculoskeletal chest pain.

Since acute chest pain can have many possible causes, a careful history and comprehensive physical examination along with inspection of the ECG and chest x-ray are mandatory in all cases where diagnostic uncertainty exists.

Risk assessment in patients with acute chest pain

Patients who present with chest pain and ischaemic ECG changes require admission and appropriate treatment. STEMI can be diagnosed quickly through characteristic ECG changes. However, ECG changes may be less obvious or absent in those with NSTEACS, which is why obtaining a good history is essential. If there is an unstable pattern of ischaemic chest pain (particularly pain at rest or lasting more than 15 minutes) admission is required for further evaluation and treatment; these patients have an ACS until proven otherwise. Troponin levels should be measured on arrival and after a further 12 hours. Patients with detectable troponin elevation are at an increased risk of early adverse cardiac events. They require prompt in-hospital treatment and continued monitoring. If the troponin levels are not elevated, patients with unstable symptoms and other high-risk features should still be investigated and treated as inpatients in the same way. Patients diagnosed with stable angina, with no elevation of troponin levels, are at lower risk of adverse cardiac events occurring early. They should be given appropriate treatment for their symptoms as well as for secondary prevention. They can then be risk stratified with functional testing such as an exercise treadmill test or with more sensitive imaging techniques such as dobutamine stress echocardiogram or myocardial perfusion scanning (e.g. via cardiac MRI or radioisotope scintigraphy).

Approximately 50 per cent of patients who present with chest pain have a non-cardiac cause; a firm alternative diagnosis may be obvious (for example, pneumothorax with an abnormal chest x-ray, or pericarditis with widespread concave ST elevation). Where the diagnosis is not obvious, patients with clear non-cardiac chest pain can be discharged once other important causes have been excluded. Patients with non-specific chest pain who have a non-diagnostic ECG and no detectable serum troponins should undergo further testing to establish or refute a diagnosis of coronary disease. Functional testing has its limitations and can give rise to false-positive results in patients without coronary disease. Conversely, patients with coronary disease may have a false-negative stress test if they have no flow-limiting coronary lesions. Newer imaging techniques using computed tomography (CT) have been used to risk-stratify patients through calcium scoring as well as CT angiography to provide further anatomical information where indicated. Recent studies of multi-slice CT have been published showing its ability to quickly identify those without coronary disease (or other conditions such as PE and aortic dissection), therefore allowing for a safe and early discharge.

INITIAL TREATMENT

Background

Patients with evolving MI often do not request medical aid until symptoms have been present for more than 1 hour. This patient delay occurs at the most critical time in the course of the illness, when pain is often severe and the risk of ventricular tachyarrhythmias and cardiac arrest is high. Therefore, any patient with chest pain suspected of having an ACS should be urgently transferred to hospital for assessment. Transfer should ideally take place by trained paramedics with cardiac monitoring and resuscitation facilities and the ability to obtain an ECG en route. Treatment and analgesia should be given en route to hospital if possible. Transmission of the ECG to the admitting hospital in advance will allow the diagnosis to be confirmed and allow for early initiation of further management.

If a patient with suspected ACS arrives in hospital, rapid processing is necessary to establish an early diagnosis and allow effective emergency care to be instituted. An appropriately trained doctor should review patients who present to the emergency department with possible ACS as soon as possible. The initial assessment should be rapid, and aimed at establishing the diagnosis, assessing the haemodynamic state and determining suitability for reperfusion therapy. Patients with clear-cut clinical features of STEMI with an ECG that demonstrates ST elevation or bundle branch block should enter a 'fast track' system, designed to ensure that they receive appropriate emergency care; any reperfusion therapy required should be instituted within 90 minutes of the initial call for medical assistance. A successful fast track system is only possible if medical staff respond rapidly to calls from the emergency department, and the aim should be to review patients with a suggestive history and ECG changes within 10 minutes of their arrival.

Emergency care

The main aims for treatment of ACS are to prevent continued ischaemia, limit myocardial damage, reduce the incidence of left ventricular dysfunction, heart failure and death. This is achieved with early identification of patients who require revascularization and treatment of complications of ischaemia including arrhythmia (VF/VT and bradycardia), heart failure and shock. Initially, in all patients with ACS, emergency care consists of symptom relief, administration of antithrombotic agents, and instigating reperfusion therapy as early as possible for STEMI.

The priorities are to:

- Establish venous access with a large-bore cannula in an arm vein providing ready access for drug administration, and institute rhythm monitoring to aid in the rapid detection and treatment of arrhythmias.

- Provide adequate analgesia, which is vital. Uncontrolled pain and anxiety are associated with sympathetic activation, with resultant detrimental effects on cardiac performance, oxygen consumption and the arrhythmia threshold. Intravenous (IV) opioids are indicated to provide rapid relief of pain. Intramuscular injections should be avoided, as they have a slower onset of action, are associated with unpredictable absorption, may cause a haematoma if thrombolytic therapy is given, and can affect CK estimations. The agent of choice is IV diamorphine 2.5–5.0 mg, given with an IV antiemetic. The dose should be repeated every 5 minutes until adequate analgesia is achieved. If repeated administration of diamorphine fails to relieve the pain, IV beta-blockers or nitrates should be considered. Respiratory depression produced by diamorphine can, if necessary, be rapidly reversed by naloxone.

- Treat pulmonary oedema with IV frusemide 40–80 mg. If pulmonary oedema is severe, an IV nitrate infusion (as detailed in Appendix A) should be commenced.

- Consider supplemental oxygen. Hypoxia is common in patients with evolving infarction, and may increase myocardial necrosis or have adverse metabolic effects. Supplemental oxygen will optimize oxygen delivery and limit ischaemia, and should be given to all patients with breathlessness or features of heart failure. Since hypoxia may be present in 20 per cent of patients with an initially uncomplicated infarct, pulse oximetry should be instituted in all cases, and oxygen given if saturation falls below 93 per cent. High-concentration (up to 60 per cent) oxygen can be given via an MC mask if necessary. If the patient has COPD, therapy with 24 or 28 per cent oxygen via a ventimask is commenced, and the concentration adjusted depending on blood gas measurements to prevent CO_2 retention in patients who are reliant on hypoxic drive to maintain ventilation.

- Commence treatment with oral antiplatelets. Aspirin (loading dose of 300 mg) and a thienopyridine (currently usually clopidogrel 600 mg, though recently published trials indicate that prasugrel 60 mg and ticagrelor may offer significant benefits). The use of clopidogrel prior to reperfusion therapy is associated with greater patency rate of the infarct-related artery and is essential for the use of stents during angioplasty.

- STEMI patients should be considered for immediate reperfusion therapy. This ideally should be primary PCI, but where this is not available, thrombolysis with fibrin-specific agents should be used.

- NSTEACS patients should be treated with low-molecular-weight heparin (LMWH) and antianginals such as beta-blockers, calcium channel antagonists and nitrates. If they are high risk, IV glycoprotein (Gp) IIb/IIIa inhibitors may be considered. They should have continuous rhythm monitoring and repeated 12-lead ECGs whilst in pain. If they develop ST elevation they should then be treated as a STEMI. If they remain in pain despite adequate treatment they should be considered for urgent coronary angiography with a view to revascularization. If the pain is continuous and severe, alternative diagnoses should be re-explored, in particular aortic dissection.

TREATMENT OF ST ELEVATION MI

Background

Prior to the advent of thrombolysis or primary PCI, the only means of achieving therapeutic reperfusion in patients with evolving MI was emergency CABG. Although no randomized trials have been performed, good results were reported for large case series from the 1970s, with an improvement in outcome compared to medically treated patients. Hospital mortality in the surgically treated patients was around 5 per cent, demonstrating that CABG can be performed in patients with evolving MI with an acceptable risk profile. With the advent of thrombolysis and primary PCI, emergency CABG is now rarely performed in patients with evolving MI, unless there is an associated early mechanical complication such as a ventricular septal rupture or acute severe mitral regurgitation. Modern reperfusion therapy has reduced mortality due to STEMI over the last three decades. Achieving reperfusion as soon as possible is fundamental to improving outcomes. Increases in time to reperfusion adversely affect early and late mortality in patients treated by either thrombolysis or primary PCI. In one study of primary PCI, there was a 7.5 per cent increase in mortality at 1 year for every 30-minute delay. Patient education therefore plays an important role in order for the symptoms to be recognized early and to call for help. Early recognition of STEMI by health care workers allows for prompt triage and initiation of reperfusion therapy at the earliest opportunity.

PRIMARY PCI

The use of primary PCI to achieve reperfusion in STEMI was first reported in 1983. Early case series suggested that primary PCI was a safe and effective means of restoring antegrade flow in the infarct-related artery (IRA) of a patient with STEMI. Potential advantages compared to thrombolysis led to a series of randomized studies comparing the two treatment modalities. Primary PCI, when performed promptly by experienced operators, has been shown to be superior to thrombolysis. A meta-analysis of 23 randomized trials with 7739 patients revealed a significantly lower rate of early death (0.7 per cent vs 0.9 per cent, $p = 0.0002$) in favour of primary PCI. Non-fatal reinfarction (3 per cent vs 7 per cent, $p < 0.0001$), and the risk of stroke (1 per cent vs 2 per cent, $p = 0.0004$) were also significantly reduced. There was an increased risk of major bleeding in the primary PCI group related to the arterial access site. This may be minimized with newer combinations of antithrombotic regimes and the use of the radial route for arterial access.

Benefits over thrombolysis

The efficacy of primary PCI is thought to predominantly result from increased patency rates achieved in the IRA (90–95 per cent with primary PCI vs 30–40 per cent with streptokinase and 50–60 per cent with fibrin-specific agents). In addition to maintaining patency, treating the underlying culprit plaque reduces rates of reinfarction and reintervention, thereby reducing overall ischaemic and mechanical complications. The lower incidence of stroke and in particular haemorrhagic stroke also contributes to the overall lower mortality in the primary PCI group. Up to 20 per cent of patients may have a contraindication to thrombolysis and in this group a significant proportion will be able to be treated by primary PCI. Finally, as successful primary PCI leads to significant reduction in myocardial damage and reduces the incidence of ischaemic complications, selected patients can be discharged earlier than if they had been treated with thrombolysis alone. Overall, compared to thrombolysis, primary PCI is cost-effective despite requiring more personnel and higher initial per treatment costs.

Assessment prior to primary PCI

Primary PCI involves arterial access, either via the femoral or radial artery and passage of a catheter to selectively engage the coronary ostia under x-ray visualization. Once the culprit vessel has been identified a small guide wire is passed along the vessel and past the occlusion. Balloons, stents and other devices can then be delivered to the point required in order to successfully treat the artery. This requires the patient to be anticoagulated, usually with unfractionated heparin, to reduce the incidence of thrombus formation on the equipment in situ.

The risk of bleeding from an angioplasty procedure should be balanced against the benefit gained. Bleeding after angioplasty, in addition to anaemia at the time of angioplasty, is associated with increased mortality. It is therefore essential that a careful history and examination identify patients at risk of bleeding and that this is communicated with the team undertaking primary PCI. This also allows for modification of the antithrombotic regime during and after the procedure.

Reactions to iodinated contrast agents are rare, however, patients with a history of allergy should be treated with IV hydrocortisone 200 mg and IV chlorpheniramine 10 mg, at the time of the procedure. A more common potential hazard is the use of contrast agents in those with renal impairment. Minimizing the amount of contrast agent used reduces the incidence as does maintaining adequate hydration. The effects of IV fluids need to be continually assessed to avoid the precipitation of fluid overload and pulmonary oedema, especially in patients with extensive anterior infarction.

Patients with complications of MI need to be identified early in order to manage them correctly. Ideally, echocardiography should be used to confirm the diagnoses of mitral regurgitation due to papillary muscle rupture, ventricular septal defect or left ventricular wall rupture. Patients in this group should be considered for urgent surgical treatment. Hypotension due to right ventricular infarct or cardiogenic shock should also be identified, as this will influence treatment during and after angioplasty.

Adjunctive therapy during primary PCI

During primary PCI various mechanical and drug therapies have been used to improve outcomes. Bare metal stents (BMS) have been shown to be superior to balloon angioplasty by reducing the risk of reocclusion and the need for reintervention due to restenosis. The CADILLAC trial compared BMS to balloon angioplasty and found significant benefits in favour of using stents including a 22.2 per cent vs 40 per cent incidence of restenosis and a 5.7 per cent vs 11.3 per cent incidence of IRA reocclusion.

Drug eluting stents (DES) have been shown to be safe in primary PCI and to reduce the need for repeat revascularization (by reducing the frequency of in-stent restenosis, ISR) when compared to BMS. Trials comparing BMS and DES in primary PCI (DEDICATION, MULTISTRATEGY and HORIZONS-AMI) have shown that DES reduce the incidence of ISR by 30–60 per cent, with no significant difference in death or stent thrombosis. Use of DES requires dual antiplatelet therapy (DAPT) to continue for 1 year whereas BMS only require 1 month. In view of the lower rate of restenosis, use of DES is preferable to BMS in smaller diameter vessels and longer lesions. However, other factors about the patient need to be considered prior to deciding on the type of stent such as the risk of bleeding, compliance with medication and the need for other long-term anticoagulents such as warfarin.

Intravenous GpIIb/IIIa inhibitors initially showed benefit for routine use in primary PCI and are still recommended routinely in many guidelines. The use of stents and higher loading doses of clopidogrel (600 mg) as well as more potent oral thienopyridines (e.g. prasugrel) have reduced the need of routine adjuvant GpIIb/IIIa in modern STEMI angioplasty. However, they should still be used in most STEMI patients where the bleeding risk is low, especially those at high risk of adverse events such as anterior infarcts and large thrombus burdens. Bivalirudin, a direct thrombin inhibitor, has shown to have a similar effect in reducing ischaemia when compared to heparin and GpIIb/IIIa (HORIZONS-AMI) trial. Its main benefit is in lower bleeding rates when angioplasty is carried out via the femoral artery. This has been demonstrated in the ACUITY trial, which assessed bleeding and outcomes in NSTEACS patients. It showed no difference in access site-related bleeding when bivalirudin was used in patients undergoing angioplasty via the radial route. There was, however, a significant reduction in bleeding when comparing the radial to femoral route (0.7 per cent vs 2.7 per cent in the GpIIb/IIIa groups) and when comparing bivalirudin to GpIIb/IIIa inhibitors in patients undergoing angioplasty via the femoral route (3 per cent vs 5.8 per cent).

Aspiration catheters are fine bore catheters which can be passed along an angioplasty wire into the IRA. They are designed to aspirate thrombus in order to reduce distal embolization. Several randomized trials have shown they improve ST-segment resolution and coronary flow. A meta-analysis of randomized trials of thrombectomy in STEMI has shown a benefit for manual aspiration catheters with a decreased combined end point of death and MI. This was largely driven by the TAPAS trial, which showed improved 30-day and 1-year survival in cases treated with routine aspiration prior to stenting, even when thrombus was not angiographically detectable.

Early discharge after primary PCI

Early discharge maintains mobility, improves quality of life and reduces the risk of hospital-acquired infection and deep vein thrombosis. Primary PCI, with use of stents and antiplatelet agents, has significantly reduced the risk of early coronary reocclusion and reinfarction after treatment for STEMI. In addition, patients can be risk stratified with regards to coronary flow at the end of the procedure and to the rest of the anatomy found at angiography. Patients who undergo successful primary PCI soon after symptom onset and who do not have any residual threatening coronary anatomy can be safely discharged early. One randomized trial (PAMI-II) has shown that early discharge of uncomplicated patients within 3 days of a primary PCI is safe and cost effective. The PAMI-II trial defined low-risk patients as: <70 years old, one or two vessel coronary disease, left ventricular ejection fraction (EF) ≥ 45 per cent, successful intervention and no malignant arrhythmia post angioplasty. The DVLA has recently changed its criteria with regards to driving and MI. Patients who have been successfully treated by primary PCI and who have an EF ≥ 40 per cent are allowed to drive after 1 week if no further intervention is planned.

THROMBOLYSIS

Background

Despite the advent of primary PCI, thrombolysis remains the initial treatment for a large proportion of acute STEMI patients in the UK. Thrombolytic therapy for acute MI was first used in 1958. Debate about its efficacy continued until 1986, when the publication of the first GISSI study clearly demonstrated the value of streptokinase. By the mid-1990s, more than 100 000 patients had been randomized into a series of large-scale thrombolytic trials, which have helped to optimize the use of thrombolytic drugs. These large-scale trials have demonstrated that:

- thrombolysis produces an important time-dependent reduction in mortality. Treatment within the first hour after symptom onset can prevent irreversible myocardial necrosis from progressing, and abort an evolving infarct. Treatment within the first 6 hours of symptom onset limits infarct size and reduces mortality by 25 per cent. Treatment between 6 and 12 hours may help to salvage some ischaemic myocardium (particularly in the border zone of the infarct) and reduces mortality by about 10 per cent. Over 12 hours from symptoms, PCI is the preferred treatment as it increases the chance of successful reperfusion and it does not carry the risks associated with late thrombolysis. Based on this first series of trials, thrombolytic therapy reduces 1-month mortality by 17 per cent, preventing 18 deaths for every 1000 patients treated. This mortality benefit is maintained in the long term, with 10-year survival rates substantially improved in treated patients. Newer, more efficacious agents have improved on these 1-month and 10-year survival figures

- mortality reduction is present regardless of age, sex or infarct site

- aspirin has an additive beneficial effect of similar magnitude to that produced by thrombolysis, and should be given to all patients with evolving MI

- the concurrent use of unfractionated heparin and thrombolytic therapy has been extensively studied. There are no beneficial effects apparent when intravenous or subcutaneous heparin is used with streptokinase or with early rt-PA (alteplase) regimens but the risk of bleeding complications is increased. For accelerated rt-PA and the newer plasminogen activators, heparin [controlled by regular activated partial thromboplastin time (aPTT) monitoring] reduces coronary reocclusion rates, and should be given for 48 hours

- thrombolysis increases the risk of stroke in the first 24 hours after treatment, but this is offset by the much larger reduction in cardiac deaths with treatment. Stroke risk is greater in older patients (over

75 years of age) and those with systolic hypertension. Bleeding from other sites can occur (particularly at the site of vascular punctures) and may require blood transfusion

- the evidence for a beneficial effect in patients with ST elevation or bundle branch block is strong. There is no clear evidence that patients with ST depression, T-wave inversion or a normal ECG derive benefit. These patients are, however, at a similar risk of bleeding complications, and should not initially receive thrombolytic therapy. For these patients, frequent or continuous ECGs should be obtained, and thrombolysis only administered if ST elevation evolves.

The benefit with thrombolysis is even more time dependent than that of primary PCI. Therefore minimizing the symptom-to-needle time is key to producing good outcomes where thrombolysis is used. If thrombolysis is the default reperfusion strategy pre-hospital thrombolysis is recommended. The CAPTIM trial compared pre-hospital thrombolysis with primary PCI in patients presenting early (<6 hour of symptoms). The composite primary end point (death, non-fatal infarction, non-fatal disabling stroke) was the same in both groups. A high proportion (85.4 per cent) of the thrombolysis group also underwent coronary early angiography, which supports the use of early adjuvant PCI in patients who have had successful thrombolysis.

Selection of thrombolytic agents

The relative efficacy of different thrombolytic agents and regimens has been compared in several trials. The early studies showed similar efficacy for streptokinase and non-accelerated rt-PA regimens. In 1993, the Global Utilization of STreptokinase for Occluded coronary arteries (GUSTO) was published. This trial demonstrated that an accelerated rt-PA regimen (given over 90 minutes rather than 3 hours) with a subsequent aPTT-controlled IV heparin infusion yielded superior IRA coronary patency rates, as well as reduced death rates. Most of the beneficial effect on mortality was obtained in patients with anterior infarction treated within 6 hours of symptom onset.

Newer plasminogen activators, produced by bioengineering techniques applied to rt-PA, have been developed to overcome disadvantages of the earlier thrombolytic agents. Fibrin-specific compounds, reteplase (r-PA) and tenecteplase (TNK), have longer half lives than the original compound, allowing for single or double bolus administration. These simplified regimens have been shown to shorten door-to-needle times.

A series of trials enrolling more than 50 000 patients (INJECT, INTIME-2, GUSTO-3, ASSENT-2) has shown that TNK has equivalent efficacy to rt-PA, whilst reteplase has at least equivalent efficacy to streptokinase. Accordingly, accelerated rt-PA or TNK with concomitant heparin are the regimens with the best record for mortality reduction. The modified plasminogen activators have the simplest dosing regimens, helping to reduce door-to-needle time.

Inclusion criteria

Where primary PCI is not available or where an additional time delay to primary PCI of 90 minutes or more is expected, thrombolysis should be given if:

- Presentation within 12 hours of onset of ischaemic cardiac pain in a patient with:
  - ST segment elevation of at least 2 mm in two adjacent chest leads
  - ST segment elevation of 1 mm in two adjacent limb leads
  - true posterior infarction or new bundle branch block.

If the presentation is >12 hours after onset of pain with ongoing symptoms and ECG evidence of evolving infarction, primary PCI should be considered first. Additionally, patients presenting with shock should be treated with primary PCI, rather than thrombolysis. The SHOCK trial showed a 20 per cent reduction in mortality at 6 months in those treated with PCI (see Cardiogenic shock).

Exclusion criteria

These continue to evolve, and are in general decreasing as our experience with thrombolytic agents increases. At present there are few absolute contraindications. Many are now regarded as relative, to be interpreted within the clinical context. Criteria include:

- known coagulation disorder, including uncontrolled anticoagulation therapy
- active peptic ulceration, varices or recent GI haemorrhage (dyspepsia alone is not a contraindication)
- severe hypertension (systolic >180 mmHg and/or diastolic >110 mmHg)
- traumatic cardiopulmonary resuscitation (CPR) (CPR performed by trained staff is not regarded as a contraindication)
- recent internal bleeding from any site (menstruation is not an absolute contraindication)
- previous haemorrhagic stroke at any time

- ischaemic stroke within the last year
- transient ischaemic attack (TIA) in last 3 months
- surgery, major trauma or head injury within the last month
- pregnancy
- diabetic retinopathy (now only a relative contraindication, as the risk of intraocular bleeding is very small and the potential benefit of thrombolysis in diabetics far outweighs this risk).

If in doubt about administering thrombolysis, a senior colleague should be consulted and if bleeding risk outweighs perceived benefits then the patient should be transferred for primary PCI, which is a safer and highly effective alternative.

Complications
Allergy
Allergic reactions to streptokinase are due to the effect of pre-existing antistreptococcal antibodies. Mild urticarial reactions are the most common allergic response, and should be treated with 200 mg IV hydrocortisone and 10 mg IV chlorpheniramine. If a more severe reaction with bronchospasm occurs, 250–500 mg of intramuscular adrenaline should be administered along with nebulized bronchodilators. Major anaphylaxis is very rare (0.1 per cent). If this occurs, with associated cardiovascular collapse, 5 mL of 1:10 000 adrenaline IV is first-line therapy, followed by rapid volume loading with IV plasma expanders, steroids and antihistamines. Allergic reactions to the newer plasminogen activators are very rare.

Haemorrhage
Minor bleeding at venepuncture sites is relatively common, but rarely requires any specific therapy other than direct compression at the site. Major haemorrhagic episodes requiring transfusion are rare. If a major bleed occurs consider the following action:

- stop thrombolytic infusion (or heparin)
- reverse heparin with protamine sulphate (10 mg per 1000 u heparin)
- give two units of fresh frozen plasma immediately
- consider the administration of tranexamic acid 10 mg/kg by slow IV injection.

Hypotension
Hypotensive reactions to thrombolytic infusion can occur with any agent, but are more common with streptokinase. They should be treated initially

by tilting the patient's head down and, in the case of streptokinase, the infusion should be slowed down or, if necessary, halted for 5 minutes. It can usually be successfully restarted when the blood pressure recovers. Atropine 0.6 mg IV can be given if a bradycardia is also present. If the hypotension persists and is clearly associated with the infusion, then the drug should be stopped, and a plasminogen activator substituted for streptokinase, as it is less likely to cause hypotension. In the case of severe persistent hypotension, fluids and inotropes can be administered cautiously if necessary.

Cerebrovascular events

The overall incidence of stroke is only minimally increased, since thrombolytic therapy causes a slight increase in cerebral haemorrhages, which is offset by a reduction in cerebral infarcts. Plasminogen activators are associated with a greater risk of haemorrhagic stroke than streptokinase. Stroke is more common in older patients. If a stroke occurs, thrombolytic or anticoagulant therapy should be discontinued. A CT scan and neurological opinion will help to determine the mechanism of the stroke and guide therapy.

Failed reperfusion

Detection and implications of failed reperfusion

Patients treated with thrombolysis who achieve effective reperfusion have a good prognosis, with hospital mortality rates of less than 5 per cent. Achievement of successful reperfusion is associated with IRA patency, restoration of rapid antegrade blood flow into a patent microcirculation and resolution of chest pain. In a substantial proportion of patients, however, reperfusion fails. In some of these patients the IRA is persistently occluded by an extensively disrupted plaque or residual thrombus. In other patients (particularly those treated late), platelet microthrombi or capillary disruption prevent reperfusion of myocardium at the tissue level despite restoration of blood flow in the epicardial IRA. Failure of reperfusion is associated with continuing chest pain, extensive infarction, electrical and haemodynamic instability, mechanical complications and a poor prognosis.

Detecting failed reperfusion in current clinical practice is based on serial evaluation of ST segments. Persistent ST elevation occurs in about one-third of patients, and is associated with failure of reperfusion, and portends an adverse prognosis. Of the 1398 patients enrolled in the INJECT trial, those with no ST resolution had a 17.5 per cent hospital mortality, those with partial resolution a 4.3 per cent mortality and those with total resolution a 2.5 per cent mortality.

Rescue angioplasty

The REACT trial as well as meta-analysis of angioplasty strategies after thrombolysis support the role of rescue angioplasty for STEMI patients who fail to reperfuse after thrombolysis. The REACT trial recruited such patients presenting within 6 hours. The criterion used to diagnose failed reperfusion was the presence of <50 per cent resolution of maximal ST elevation on the 90-minute post-thrombolysis ECG. The original trial showed a significant reduction in reinfarction at 6 months in those undergoing rescue angioplasty when compared to repeat thrombolysis or conservative therapy (2.1 per cent vs 10.5 per cent vs 8.5 per cent). Follow-up data at 1 year showed a sustained benefit with increased event-free survival in the rescue PCI group. Accordingly, all patients should have an ECG recorded 90 minutes after commencing thrombolysis. Patients who have less than 50 per cent ST segment resolution in the infarct zone should be considered for rescue angioplasty.

Recurrent ischaemia and early PCI after thrombolysis

Following successful thrombolytic therapy, patients are often left with a residual high grade stenosis or an 'inflamed' ruptured plaque. Recurrent ischaemia occurs in up to one-third of thrombolyzed patients, and is associated with increased hospital mortality. Usually, early recurrent ischaemia is related to further thrombus formation at the site of the original unstable atherosclerotic plaque. The GRACIA-1 trial looked at patients who were successfully thrombolysed and compared routine angiography within 24 hours with an ischaemia-guided approach. Among the subjects undergoing early angiography, stenting of the IRA was performed in 80 per cent. This was associated with a significant reduction in a combined end point of death, reinfarction or revascularization (9 per cent vs 21 per cent at 12 months). Index hospital stay was also significantly reduced in the early group.

Recently, another trial (TRANSFER-AMI) of 1059 patients compared immediate transfer for PCI after thrombolysis (with tenecteplase) with standard treatment with rescue angioplasty if required. Angiography was undertaken at a median of 2.8 hours in the immediate transfer group and 32.5 hours in the standard treatment group. In the standard group, 34.9 per cent underwent early angioplasty for rescue, shock and reinfarction. Overall, early angiography was associated with significantly reduced recurrent ischaemia (0.2 per cent vs 2.1 per cent), as well as a reduced combined end point of death, reinfarction, recurrent ischaemia, new or worsening heart failure or cardigenic shock within 30 days.

Trials of 'facilitated' angioplasty (where angioplasty is performed immediately after pharmacological treatment such as thrombolysis) have shown significantly worse results compared to primary PCI; this is due to an increase in bleeding and ischaemic events. For example, the ASSENT-4 trial demonstrated a higher in-hospital mortality for facilitated PCI (after thrombolysis with tenecteplase) compared to primary PCI (6 per cent vs 3 per cent), causing early termination of the trial.

The higher ischaemic events were put down to suboptimal antithrombotic treatment after thrombolysis and the fact that thrombolysis itself leads to a pro-thrombotic state. The higher incidence of bleeding in the facilitated group also contributed to the higher mortality.

Overall, the data suggest that early angiography should be performed following successful thrombolysis, although very early intervention carries an increased risk of adverse events. A reasonable approach would be to transfer the patient to an angioplasty centre as soon as practically possible with a view to angiography within 24 hours. This strategy would also allow for earlier invervention in the event of patients developing recurrent ischaemia or reinfarction.

STEMI with normal coronary arteries

Up to 20 per cent of patients with clinical features of STEMI may have normal coronary arteries. Conditions which classically mimic STEMI include myocarditis, takotsubo cardiomyopathy and coronary spasm. In addition, thromboembolic disease may produce a temporary thrombotic occlusion similar to that of classical STEMI. Therefore, it is important to investigate further those patients who present without the usual risk factors for STEMI. The function of the left ventricle should be assessed in all patients with STEMI who turn out to have normal coronary arteries preferably with cardiac MRI. This is the most sensitive way to detect if myocardial damage is due to an ischaemic or myocarditic process by the pattern of scarring on late gadolinium enhancement. Patients with thrombotic occlusion with no evidence of coronary disease should be investigated for a right to left shunt, commonly a patent foramen ovale or secundum atrial septal defect. This can be undertaken by contrast echocardiography with agitated saline. Takotsubo (or stress) cardiomyopathy is a diagnosis almost exclusive to females and occurs is association with severe stress such as recent bereavement. Patients present with signs and symptoms exactly that of acute STEMI; however, they have patent coronary arteries with characteristic ballooning of the left ventricular apex. This recovers in all cases within 6 weeks; however, there is a risk or arrhythmia, shock and death within the first few days of presentation.

TREATMENT OF NON-ST ELEVATION ACS

The management of NSTEACS is different from that of acute STEMI. Treatment is aimed at reducing persistent ischaemia and the risk of reinfarction as opposed to opening an occluded artery to abort an infarction. Medical therapy has limited impact on mortality but does lead to a reduction in subsequent infarction and persistent ischaemia by stabilizing coronary plaques. The addition of coronary angiography provides anatomical information on the culprit lesion, the extent of disease, global and regional left ventricular function and provides a starting point for subsequent revascularization. In deciding which patients should undergo early intervention, the risks of the procedure (bleeding, renal failure, stroke) have to be balanced against the risk from further ischaemia. This can be difficult, as often the patients at highest risk of complications are also at the highest risk of further ischaemia. Furthermore, there is a wide heterogeneity of patients presenting with an ACS. The initial assessment of risk is thus central to the decisions made regarding a conservative or invasive strategy and this should be made on presentation of the patient to the accident and emergency department. Although most patients stabilize with aggressive antianginal therapy, 50–60 per cent of patients still go on to have 'failure' of therapy, either defined as further ischaemia at rest or on early exercise testing.

The characteristics that increase the likelihood of failure of medical therapy are:

- reversible ST segment change
- previous angina
- prior aspirin use
- family history of premature coronary disease
- increased age.

If all these characteristics are present, medical failure occurs in 90 per cent of cases. If none is present, the majority of patients settle with medical therapy.

Clinical features and the 12-lead ECG

The medical history and physical examination provide some help for risk stratification. Patients with multiple risk factors for vascular disease are at increased risk of adverse events. Older age and previous aspirin use are also markers of adverse risk. A highly unstable pattern of symptoms with recent rest pain is also an adverse risk factor. Evidence of haemodynamic instability or compromise indicates a poor prognosis.

The PRAIS-UK study was a registry of 1061 patients admitted to 56 hospitals in the UK, half of whom had immediate access to angiography. From this study, the 6-month risk of death or MI was estimated and stratified according to age, ECG changes and the presence of heart failure. Compared to subjects aged <60 years, the relative risk was 2.1 for those aged 60–70, and 2.8 for those over 70 years. The registry also confirmed the value of the ECG in determining risk: compared to having a normal ECG, documented ECG T-wave inversion and ST-segment depression increased the relative risk of events at 6 months by three-fold and five-fold, respectively. The presence of heart failure increased risk by 1.9, similar to the two-fold risk of being male. In another study, sequential risk for death or MI at 12-month follow-up was evaluated in 911 patients with unstable angina or non-Q-wave MI. The risk with a normal ECG, T-wave inversion, ST elevation, ST depression and both ST depression and elevation was 8 per cent, 13 per cent, 15 per cent, 17 per cent and 25 per cent, respectively. The duration of the ischaemia also has a bearing on outcome. Episodes of ischaemia that are associated with ST segment change and persist for 10 minutes or more are associated with the worse prognosis.

Based on these data, a successful algorithm has been developed to triage patients with acute, ischaemic-sounding chest pain. The primary ECG abnormality necessitating admission was ST-segment depression or elevation greater than 1 mm. In the presence of lesser changes such as

- ST elevation 0.5–1 mm
- ST depression 0.25–1 mm
- T-wave inversion in >2 leads
- Q waves
- left ventricular hypertrophy
- abnormal rhythm

a diagnosis of cardiac chest pain was considered likely if the patient was male, or if pain radiated to the neck or left arm, or if there was associated nausea/sweating, or if the patient reported a history of ischaemic heart disease. Where the ECG was normal, three or more of these latter features would be required to increase suspicion of an ACS.

RISK SCORES IN NSTEACS

Fundamental to the development of modern risk scores in NSTEACS is the quantification of serum troponin. As described earlier, troponin measurement is now the gold standard test for detection of myocardial injury. In ACS, troponin levels rise about 4 hours after the onset of chest pain in 30–50 per cent of patients with 100 per cent of infarct patients being positive at 12 hours. In a review of 4000 patients with acute ischaemic syndromes, troponin T levels were raised in 33 per cent of patients. A strong relationship exists between the level of peak plasma troponin at 12 hours from the onset of pain and the extent of myocardial damage.

Furthermore, several studies have demonstrated that the absolute levels of troponin have a strong relationship to clinical outcome such as death and MI over the short- and medium-term period after presentation with an ACS. In an early trial of 112 patients with unstable anginal symptoms, death or MI occurred in 30 per cent of those with an elevated troponin T (>0.2 µg/L), compared to 2 per cent in the remainder. In the larger GUSTO-IIa trial, troponin T elevation was confirmed to strongly predict 30-day mortality. Similarly, troponin I elevation was related to mortality in ACS: in a study published in 1996, mortality at 42 days was 1.0 per cent with a troponin I level <0.4 µg/L compared to 7.5 per cent with a troponin I level >9.0 µg/L (Figure 1.6). In the FRISC study, 963 patients participating in a randomized study of LMWH (dalteparin) in unstable angina had troponin T measured. A total of 766 patients had a pre-discharge exercise test. Cardiac death or MI at 5-month follow-up occurred in 5 per cent, 9 per cent and 13 per cent of patients with a maximum troponin level of 0.06 µg/L, 0.06–0.2 µg/L, and >0.2 µg/L at 12 hours, respectively. Similarly, exercise tolerance and ST-segment depression stratified patients into low, intermediate and high risk with death/MI in 5 per cent, 13 per cent and 29 per cent, respectively. Combination of the two variables (troponin T and exercise test) predicted adverse outcome in 1 per cent of low risk, 7 per cent of intermediate risk and 20 per cent of high-risk patients (Figure 1.7). Thus, elevation of cardiac troponin indicates the presence of minor myocyte damage, which is associated with a high risk of subsequent progression to MI and death in patients with unstable angina.

Risk assessment can be further refined using clinical scoring systems which have been developed from the analysis of large cohorts of patients with NSTEACS. They use features from the history, clinical examination, ECG changes and biomarkers to predict the risk of further events. The most sensitive for predicting events in hospital and up to 6 months is the GRACE score (http://www.outcomes.org/grace/). The TIMI risk score for

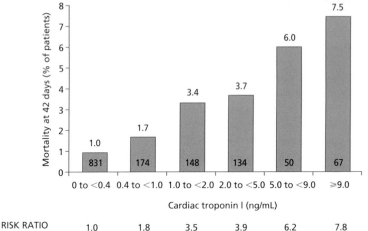

| RISK RATIO | 1.0 | 1.8 | 3.5 | 3.9 | 6.2 | 7.8 |
| 95% CONFIDENCE INTERVAL | — | 0.5–6.7 | 1.2–10.6 | 1.3–11.7 | 1.7–22.3 | 2.6–23.0 |

Figure 1.6 Mortality rates at 42 days according to the level of cardiac Troponin I measured at enrolment. (Reproduced with permission from Antman et al. (1996) Copyright © 1996 Massachusetts Medical Society. All rights reserved.)

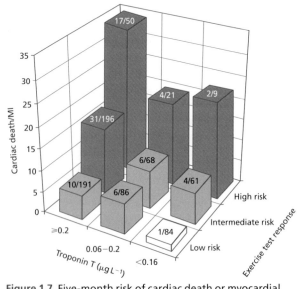

Figure 1.7 Five-month risk of cardiac death or myocardial infarction (MI) in relation to exercise test response and maximal troponin T levels during the first 24 hours. (Reproduced with permission from Lindahl et al. (1997))

NSTEACS is simpler to use though it is less accurate at predicting events than GRACE. However, it has an added advantage in that it is the only scoring system that has been shown to identify patients with a long-term benefit of an early invasive treatment strategy in a randomized trial. It assigns one point to each of the following risk factors:

- age ≥ 65
- three or more risk factors for coronary artery disease (family history/diabetes/current smoker/hyperlidaemia/hypertension)
- known coronary stenosis ≥50 per cent
- aspirin use in the preceding 7 days
- two or more episodes of severe angina during the previous 24 hours
- ST segment deviation on ECG of ≥0.5 mm
- elevated serum cardiac biomakers.

The score predicts the recurrence of ischaemia within 14 days: 0–1 = 4.7 per cent, 2 = 8.3 per cent, 3 = 13.2 per cent, 4 = 19.9 per cent, 5 = 26.2 per cent, 6 = 40.9 per cent. Patients with a score of 3 or more are considered high risk and are likely to benefit from an early invasive strategy, especially if their biomarkers are positive.

High-risk patients

The American Heart Association/American College of Cardiology (AHA/ACC) guidelines recommend an invasive strategy in NSTEACS in the following situations:

- recurrent angina/ischaemia at rest or low-level exercise despite intensive medical therapy
- signs or symptoms of heart failure or new or worsening mitral regurgitation
- high-risk findings on non-invasive stress testing
- reduced left ventricular function (EF <40 per cent)
- haemodynamic instability
- sustained ventricular tachycardia (VT)
- PCI within the previous 6 months
- prior CABG
- high-risk score (e.g. TIMI or GRACE)
- new or presumably new ST-segment depression
- elevated cardiac biomarkers (troponin I and T).

Patients with recent PCI are likely to have a restenosis or stent thrombosis best treated with reintervention. Prior CABG represents another subgroup where early intervention is of benefit due to the high rate of venous graft failure. Patients with reduced left ventricular function, acute heart failure or previous anterior Q-wave MIs have sufficient risk to support a policy of early angiography. Patients with extensive co-morbidities and patients with chest pain with low-risk scores are unlikely to benefit from an invasive strategy.

Low-risk patients

Non-invasive stress testing with a low-level treadmill exercise test (two stages of the Bruce protocol) should be performed in patients free of ischaemia at rest or on minimal exertion for 12–24 hours. Should patients be discharged prior to this, symptom-limited exercise testing may be done within 7–10 days of presentation.

Where the baseline ECG has resting ST-segment depression (>0.1 mV), bundle branch block, left ventricular hypertrophy, an intraventricular conduction defect, a paced rhythm, or the patient is on digoxin therapy, stress perfusion imaging (radioisotope or MRI) or stress echocardiography may be done to identify a substrate for ischaemia. Those that subsequently have a positive stress test should undergo coronary angiography with a view to revascularization.

REVASCULARIZATION STRATEGIES IN NSTEACS

PCI has become the established treatment for NSTEACS. The adjunctive use of intracoronary stents and GpIIb/IIIa inhibitors has diminished the risk and improved the outcome associated with PCI. At present, the rate of in-hospital mortality is still less than 1 per cent, with indicators of infarction risk well defined in clinical and angiographic terms.

Historically, in unstable angina, CABG surgery has been associated with an increased operative mortality at 3.7 per cent (much improved in FRISC-II with an in-hospital mortality of 1.2 per cent) with predictors of risk being left ventricular dysfunction, the need for pre-bypass intra-aortic balloon pumping, and a history of previous CABG. With successful hospital discharge, the 5-year survival is 90 per cent with the greatest relative benefit seen in those with reduced left ventricular function – in one study in patients with a left ventricular EF <50 per cent, the 3-year mortality was 6.1 per cent in patients after surgery, compared to 17.6 per cent in medically treated patients.

The FRISC-II study compared an early invasive and conservative strategy in 2457 patients with unstable angina. The patients were of mean age 66 years (70 per cent men). Angiography was performed within 7 days in 96 per cent of the invasive group compared to only 10 per cent of the conservative group. Revascularization (55 per cent PCI, 45 per cent CABG) was performed within 10 days in 71 per cent of the invasive group compared to 9 per cent of the conservative group, and within 6 months in 77 per cent and 37 per cent, respectively. At 6-month follow-up, the invasive group had a 22 per cent (9.4 per cent vs 12.1 per cent, p = 0.031) reduction in the composite end point of death/MI through a reduction in the rate of MI. Furthermore, there was a reduction in readmission rate by 44 per cent, as well as a 36 per cent reduction in the presence of angina compared to the conservative group. The benefits were sustained to 5 years: the primary end point of death or MI was reduced by 19 per cent, and there was a 27 per cent reduction in the rate of MI alone in the invasive group. The FRISC-II study also randomized patients to treatment with and without the LMWH dalteparin. The benefit of the adjunctive use of dalteparin was seen in the conservative group with a reduction in primary end point, although it had no additional effect on the invasive arm.

The TACTICS-TIMI 18 trial also compared an early invasive and conservative strategy in patients with NSTEACS who were given the GpIIb/IIIa inhibitor tirofiban. Over half the patients had elevated troponin T levels and 48 per cent had ECG changes present, indicating a high-risk population. Almost all (97 per cent) of the invasive group underwent coronary angiography at a median time of 22 hours after randomization. Revascularization was undertaken in 61 per cent of patients in the early invasive arm (41 per cent PCI, 20 per cent CABG). In the conservative arm, 51 per cent underwent angiography during the initial hospitalization with 37 per cent undergoing revascularization. This resulted in a significant reduction in death and non-fatal MI in the invasive group of 35 per cent at 1 month (4.7 per cent vs 7 per cent, p = 0.02) and 26 per cent at 6 months (7.3 per cent vs 9.5 per cent, p < 0.05). Subanalysis also showed that those with a TIMI risk score of ≥3 or a troponin T of ≥ 0.1ng/ml gained the most from an invasive strategy, whereas those with a score of ≤2 or troponin T of ≤0.1ng/ml had similar outcomes with either strategy.

The RITA-3 study also showed benefit for an invasive strategy with reduced refractory angina at 4 months (4.4 per cent vs 9.3 per cent). There was no reduction in death or MI at 1 year, but analysis of the 5-year follow-up data has shown a reduction of 26 per cent (p = 0.03) in cardiovascular death and MI. When stratified according to risk, the patients in the highest risk group appeared to benefit the most from intervention.

A meta-analysis of seven trials involving 8375 NSTEACS (including RITA-3, TACTICS-TIMI 18 and FRISC II) patients showed a significant benefit in survival at 2 years in those treated with early intervention (all-cause mortality 4.9 per cent vs 6.5 per cent, p = 0.001).

With regards to timing of intervention, several trials have assessed early vs delayed intervention. The ISAR-COOL trial was a small (401 patients), double-centre study in which NSTEACS patients were randomized to early intervention or prolonged antithrombotic treatment followed by intervention. The median time to intervention was 2.4 hours for early intervention and 86 hours in the antithrombotic arm. Early intervention showed a significant benefit in reducing non-fatal MI or death at 30 days (5.9 per cent vs 11.6 per cent, p = 0.04), which was attributed mainly to events whilst awaiting catheterization. The more recent TIMACS trial involving 3031 patients compared early (≤24 hours) vs delayed (≥36 hours) intervention. The median time to intervention was 14 hours in the early arm and 50 hours in the delayed group. Follow-up at 6 months revealed no difference in the primary end-point of death, MI or stroke. However, there was a reduction in refractory ischaemia in the early invasive group.

Overall, high-risk patients, without contraindications to intervention, should undergo an early invasive strategy ideally within 24 hours of presentation, and those patients with ongoing ischaemia despite optimal medical therapy should be considered for more immediate revascularization. Patients who are high risk with positive troponin should receive GpIIb/IIIa inhibitors in the catheter laboratory. Up-front use of GpIIb/IIIa inhibitors is recommended in many guidelines but routine use is associated with a signficantly increased risk of bleeding and the benefits in reducing ischaemia are mainly conferred at the time of PCI (see Glycoprotein IIb/IIIa inhibitors).

BLEEDING RISK IN ACS

Successful treatment of ACS involves the use of potent antithrombotic regimens allied with PCI. Unfortunately, bleeding is the most common non-cardiac complication associated with coronary intervention. The use of antithrombotic agents increases the risk of both access site-related bleeding, and non-access site-related bleeds such as gastrointestinal, cerebral and retroperitoneal haemorrhage. There is a strong association between bleeding and adverse events with risks increased by five-fold for MI, four-fold for death and three-fold for stroke at 30 days. The mechanisms for this are mutifactorial including haemodynamic effects, the cessation of antithrombotic drugs, and, possibly, adverse effects from blood transfusion. Bleeding is also commoner among older, more frail subjects with significant co-morbidities, who are also at higher risk of ischaemic events. Therefore the benefit gained from treatment has to balanced against the risks of bleeding and treatment needs to be tailored to individual patients. Several risk scores have been developed to predict the risks of bleeding in an effort to assist with the decision-making. The CRUSADE score (http://www.crusadebleedingscore.org/) was developed from a registry of 89 000 patients to predict the risk of in-hospital bleeding in NSTEACS. More recently another system from over 302 000 patients who underwent PCI has been developed, which assigns points to the following nine variables:

ACS type	STEMI 10 points/NSTEACS 3 points
Cardiogenic shock	8 points
Female gender	6 points
Previous congestive heart failure	5 points
No previous PCI	4 points
NHYA class IV heart failure	4 points
Peripheral vascular disease	2 points
Age: 66–75 – 2 points/76–85 – 5 points/≥85	8 points
Renal function	1 point for every 10 unit decrease in eGFR if <90

The risk of bleeding on the current admission was classed as low if scores were ≤7, medium 8–17 and high ≥18 with prevalence of 0.63 per cent, 1.8 per cent and 5 per cent respectively.

Vascular access complications can be minimized by using the radial rather than femoral route. GI bleeding has been shown to be reduced by the use of gastroprotective medication in high-risk patients. Careful dosing of LMWH and unfractionated heparin (UFH) is required in those with renal impairment. Similarly, in patients at high risk of bleeding, the use of alternative agents can be considered. These agents are as effective as heparin and GpIIb/IIIa inhibitors at reducing ischaemic events while benefiting from lower rates of bleeding. These agents include bivalirudin, which can be used alone in patients undergoing intervention, and fondaparinux, which can be used alone in those being managed medically, or with heparin among those undergoing intervention.

Thrombocytopenia

Thrombocytopenia can occur after treatment for ACS as a result of exposure to heparins or GpIIb/IIIa inhibitors. Heparin-induced thrombocytopenia (HIT), is a serious, immunoglobulin-mediated complication that often leads to thromboembolic complications. It occurs with UFH (incidence 5 per cent) and LMWH (incidence 0.5 per cent) usually after between 5 and 10 days of use (or sooner if there has been previous exposure to heparins), and is associated with a 50 per cent reduction in the platelet count or a drop to $< 100 \times 10^9$ platelets/L. It should be treated with the cessation of heparin and introduction of another antithrombotic agent such as lepirudin or danaparoid. Bleeding complications of HIT are rare but 50 per cent of patients with HIT develop arterial or venous thrombosis which can be life threatening. Further exposure to heparins should be avoided in patients who have had HIT.

GpIIb/IIIa-induced thrombocytopenia is often more profound with platelet counts of $< 50 \times 10^9$ platelets/L. It occurs more frequently with abciximab (up to 2.4 per cent) and less with eptifibatide (0.2 per cent) and tirofiban (0.5 per cent). The GpIIb/IIIa inhibitor and heparin should be discontinued. Most patients remain asymptomatic and platelet counts begin to improve within 24 hours. Platelet transfusions should be reserved for those with bleeding. Thrombosis is rare with GpIIb/IIIa inhibitor-induced thrombocytopenia; however, there is a higher incidence of adverse events, due to bleeding, repeat revascularization, recurrent ischaemia and death.

ADJUNCTIVE MEDICAL THERAPY

Aspirin

Unless there is a contradidication, aspirin should be administered to all patients with NSTEACS and STEMI at presentation. It should be continued indefinitely in all patients with suspected or proven coronary disease. Aspirin inhibits the cyclooxygenase enzyme in platelets which leads to the formation of thromboxane A_2, a potent stimulus to platelet activation. Data from the Veterans Administration Cooperative Study, the

Canadian Multicenter Trial and the Montreal Heart Institute Study confirmed that the use of aspirin in unstable angina reduced the risk of cardiac death and non-fatal MI by 51–72 per cent. From a meta-analysis of seven antiplatelet studies, a 35 per cent reduction in vascular events occurred over 20 months with aspirin. The body of evidence suggests that aspirin should be initiated at a dose of either 160 or 325 mg in patients not already receiving aspirin with subsequent daily dosing at 75–325 mg. With aspirin, however, only one pathway of platelet activation is inhibited and the platelet may also be readily activated by adenosine diphosphate (ADP), thrombin and collagen. Aspirin reduces platelet aggregation, enhancing recanalization in STEMI, and reducing the risk of further vascular events in patients with previous MI. The effect of aspirin on mortality in patients with acute MI has been studied in 15 trials, enrolling more than 19 000 patients (most of these patients were enrolled in ISIS-2). Overall mortality with aspirin therapy is reduced by around 20 per cent. This benefit is maintained with continued treatment over several years. A loading dose of 150 mg produces rapid and complete inhibition of thromboxane-mediated platelet inhibition. For long-term treatment, higher doses are more gastrotoxic. A dose of 75 mg/day maintains virtually complete long-term cyclooxygenase inhibition, and is suitable for chronic therapy.

There are few contraindications to the use of aspirin, but it should not be given to patients with:

- known hypersensitivity to aspirin
- bleeding peptic ulcer
- coagulation disorder
- severe hepatic disease.

There is no clear evidence of a relationship between effectiveness and time from onset of symptoms, and aspirin should immediately be given to all patients diagnosed to have evolving or recent ACS, even if presentation is late. In patients who do not tolerate aspirin through hypersensitivity or major gastrointestinal intolerance, a thienopyridine should be considered.

Clopidogrel
Clopidogrel is a thienopyridine which blocks ADP-mediated platelet aggregation and the activation of the GpIIb/IIIa receptor, which cross-links platelets through fibrinogen. It was shown to be of value in NSTEACS in the CURE trial: this randomized 12 562 patients with NSTEACS

non-cardiac surgery or who have a bleed, the cessation of antiplatelets should be discussed with a cardiologist first.

Anticoagulants

As previously discussed, heparin is required for 48 hours after thrombolysis with plasminogen activators. Heparin is not beneficial and is not recommended as routine therapy after streptokinase. UFH was used in the initial trials of plasminogen activators, however more recently the EXTRACT-TIMI 25 trial showed that the use of LMWH post thrombolysis resulted in a lower rate of reinfarction compared to UFH (9.9 per cent vs 12 per cent, p = 0.001) at a cost of increased major bleeding (2.1 per cent vs 1.4 per cent, p < 0.001). In meta-analyses, the use of LMWH has been shown to be more effective than UFH in reducing reinfarction and ischaemia in NSTEACS treated medically with no increase in bleeding. In the SYNERGY trial, LMWH has also been shown to be as effective as UFH in patients undergoing an early invasive strategy albeit at an increased risk of major bleeding (9.9 per cent vs 7.6 per cent). The increased risk of bleeding in patients undergoing PCI may have been due to the addition of UFH while the previous dose of LMWH was still active. In the STACKENOX trial the addition of UFH to enoxaparin resulted in a considerable and prolonged increase in clotting parameters (anti-Xa and anti-IIa) but had no effect on the more routinely measured activated clotting time (ACT). Additionally, LMWH alone during PCI in the STEEPLE trial showed lower rates of mainly femoral access site complications. However, the use of UFH is still recommended during PCI procedures as it is rapidly effective with a measurable change in the ACT and it can be promptly reversed with protamine if necessary.

Bivalirudin, a direct thrombin inhibitor, is also effective in STEMI and NSTEACS patients and can be continued during PCI. The main advantage of bivalirudin is the reduction in bleeding compared to the use of heparin and GpIIb/IIIa inhibitors. In NSTEACS, fondaparinux, a factor Xa inhibitor, when given subcutaneously at a dose of 2.5 mg, was shown to be as effective as the LMWH enoxaparin in the OASIS-5 trial. Major bleeds were reduced by 48 per cent in the fondaparinux group, although it was noted that there was a higher incidence of catheter-related thrombus which did not impact on the primary end point. Therefore fondaparinux can be recommended for NSTEACS, particularly for those at high risk of bleeding, when intervention is likely to be delayed, or when medical management is preferred. If patients on fondaparinux undergo PCI, it is recommended that they receive heparin during the procedure. Fondaparinux was also studied in STEMI in the OASIS-6 trial involving 12 092 patients either treated with thrombolysis, primary PCI or without any reperfusion therapy. There was a significant reduction in the primary end point of death or reinfarction at 30 days when compared to UFH. (9.7 per cent vs 11.2 per cent, $p = 0.008$). This benefit was mainly observed among patients who were not treated with primary PCI. Even those that did not receive reperfusion therapy without a conventional indication for UFH benefited from fondaparinux in reducing the incidence of the primary end point. The benefits were onserved without an increase in bleeding and stroke.

Overall, anticoagulants are recommended in all patients with ACS, but the doses and agents used need to be carefully considered in relation to patients' bleeding risks.

Glycoprotein IIB/IIIA inhibitors

Background

Because activation of the GpIIb/IIIa receptor is the final common pathway of platelet aggregation through its ability to cross-link with other GpIIb/IIIa receptors through fibrinogen or von Willebrand factor, different agents have been developed specifically to inhibit this process. These are the chimeric (murine–human) antibody fragment to the GpIIb/IIIa receptor, abciximab (Reopro™), synthetic peptides such as eptifibatide (Integrelin™) and synthetic non-peptides such as tirofiban (Aggrastat™). Abciximab is a F_{ab} antibody fragment of a human–murine (chimeric) monoclonal antibody (c7E3) with a short plasma half-life but with a strong receptor affinity, persisting for weeks (although platelet aggregation returns to normal within 48 hours). Abciximab is relatively non-specific and also inhibits the vitronectin ($\alpha_v\beta_3$) receptor which is on endothelial cells and the MAC-1 receptor on leucocytes. By contrast, the synthetic (small molecule) GpIIb/IIIa inhibitors have half-lives of 2–3 hours and are more specific to the receptor. There is an increased risk of bleeding with these agents, which is typically mucocutaneous or at access sites, particularly at the site of a femoral artery sheath.

Abciximab (Reopro™)

Abciximab has the most data among the GpIIb/IIIa inhibitors, in particular when used after angiography. Analysis of pooled data from three large trials (EPIC/EPILOG/EPISTENT) including 7290 patients with ACS receiving stenting has shown a 29 per cent reduction in late mortality when compared to placebo. Based on the experience of the EPIC trial, the EPILOG trial confirmed the need to reduce the bolus heparin dosing to

70 U/kg during intervention to diminish this risk. More recent data from the ISAR-REACT 2 study have shown the benefit for abciximab in addition to loading with clopidogrel 600 mg in NSTEACS. At 30 days, the composite end point of death/MI/urgent target vessel revascularization was reduced in the abciximab group by 25 per cent, compared to placebo (8.9 per cent vs 11.9 per cent, p = 0.03). Subgroup analysis had revealed that the benefits were isolated to those patients who had positive troponins. Interestingly, the 1-year follow-up of ISAR-REACT 2 has shown continued benefit in the primary end point (23.3 per cent vs 28 per cent, p = 0.012), which now also extended to troponin-negative patients.

The use of abciximab up-front (prior to angiography) has been studied in a meta-analysis of 29 570 patients. The benefit of abciximab was only observed in patients who subsequently went on to have PCI. Based on current evidence, abciximab should be considered in the catheter laboratory for all troponin-positive NSTEACS requiring PCI. Among STEMI patients, the use of abciximab has been shown to be of benefit in a large meta-analysis with 27 115 patients. However, several of the trials did not use stents, and none of the included studies used the higher loading dose of clopidogrel, so these studies do not really reflect contemporary practice. Indeed, a more recent study, BRAVE-3, showed no additional benefit on infarct size (measured by single-photon emission CT) with abciximab when 600 mg of clopidogrel was used. Based on the evidence, the use of abciximab for STEMI is recommended, but not mandated, and may be reserved for patients at low bleeding risk, who have not received adequate loading with clopidogrel, or those with a large thrombus burden.

Tirofiban and eptifibatide

The small molecues tirofiban and eptifibatide have also been shown to be of benefit when used in NSTEACS.

In the PRISM study, treatment with tirofiban in addition to aspirin and UFH reduced death and non-fatal MI at 7 days (4.9 per cent vs 8.3 per cent, p < 0.01) and 30 days (8.7 per cent vs 11.9 per cent, p < 0.01). Benefit was restricted to those patients who were troponin positive. In a concurrent trial, PRISM-PLUS, 1915 patients with NSTEACS received either tirofiban alone, tirofiban with heparin or heparin alone (all with aspirin) for a mean of 71 hours. The tirofiban-alone group had an excess of mortality and was discontinued. Angiography was done as clinically indicated. Administration of tirofiban with heparin yielded significantly lower 7-day and 6-month composite end points (death/MI/refractory ischaemia) compared to heparin alone, 12.9 per cent vs 17.9 per cent (32 per cent reduction, p < 0.01) and 27.7 per cent vs 32.1 per cent (a 19 per cent reduction, p < 0.05), respectively. Tirofiban was compared to abciximab in the TARGET study and was found to be inferior at 30 days with regards to the primary end point of death, MI and urgent revascularization. However, there was no significant difference at 6 months and 1 year follow-up.

Eptifibatide is a cyclic heptapeptide that contains the KGD (lysine-glycine-aspartate) amino acid sequence. In the PURSUIT trial, 10 948 patients with NSTEACS received heparin, low dose, or high-dose eptifibatide (Integrilin™) for 72 hours. At 30 days, the composite end point of death/non-fatal MI was significantly lower in the eptifibatide group, driven by a 14.2 per cent vs 15.7 per cent (p < 0.05) in the eptifibatide and placebo group, respectively. This occurred through a non-significant reduction in MI. The ESPRIT study looked at patients undergoing PCI with a stent (46 per cent with NSTEACS) and compared eptifibatide to placebo. The primary end point was a composite of death, MI, urgent target vessel revascularization and thrombotic bailout GpIIb/IIIa inhibitor therapy within 48 hours after randomization. It showed a reduction in the eptifibatide arm from 10.5 per cent to 6.6 per cent (p = 0.0015) which was sustained to 6 months.

The up-front use of these two agents is recommended in NSTEACS. However, early angiography is becoming more widely available, and allows for PCI to relieve ischaemia. The use of GpIIb/IIIa inhibitors after angiography has the added advantage of selecting the patients likely to benefit the most (i.e. those undergoing PCI), and avoids administration to subjects requiring surgical revascularization, or to those at an increased risk of bleeding. This was shown to be the case in the EARLY-ACS trial where up-front eptifibatide was compared to delayed provisional use. There was no difference in the primary end point (death/MI/recurrent ischaemia requiring urgent revascularization/thrombotic bailout). However, there was a significant risk of major bleeding (2.5 per cent vs 1.8 per cent, p = 0.015).

Compared with abciximab, there are fewer data supporting the use of the small molecules in STEMI. The EVA-AMI and MULTISTRATEGY studies compared abciximab with eptifibatide and tirofiban, respectively. Both trials showed similar benefits with the smaller molecules to abciximab. However, as with abciximab, the benefit in addition to higher loading doses of clopidogrel has not been shown. In the ON-TARGET 2 trial, early tirofiban was used with 600 mg of clopidogrel and was not found to have any clinical benefit compared to placebo. Overall, the small molecules can be recommended for selective use in NSTEACS, but there is not enough data to recommend their routine use in STEMI.

Beta-blockers

Beta-blockers have antiarrhythmic, anti-ischaemic and antihypertensive properties. Small studies indicate that these beneficial effects reduce chest pain, myocardial wall stress and infarct size in patients with STEMI. An overview of almost 30 000 patients randomized to placebo or IV therapy in the pre-thrombolytic era indicated that they were well tolerated, preserved left ventricular function and reduced the incidence of arrhythmia and early mortality.

The large COMMIT study compared the use of early IV then oral metoprolol with placebo in STEMI patients. The metoprolol group showed a modest reduction in reinfarction and ventricular fibrillation but no overall benefit on mortality. More importantly, the rate of cardiogenic shock was significantly higher in the metoprolol group. Therefore, routine use of intravenous beta-blockers cannot be recommended for all patients with STEMI. As maximum mortality benefit from beta-blocker therapy is obtained in higher-risk patients, whose infarctions are complicated by arrhythmias or heart failure; treatment should be directed to specific problems such as ongoing chest pain, poorly controlled hypertension and tachy-arrhythmia. However, patients should be carefully selected to avoid those at risk of developing shock (e.g. patients with large, un-reperfused anterior infarcts and patients with mechanical complications).

Long-term oral beta-blockers, commenced in the convalescent phase of MI, have been evaluated in a large number of placebo-controlled trials. In a recent meta-analysis of 82 trials enrolling more than 54 000 patients, mortality was reduced by almost 25 per cent due to the prevention of reinfarction and sudden death. These benefits are apparent irrespective of age, site of infarction, and presence or absence of previous MI or complications. Serious side effects are rare. Benefit is still apparent after several years of therapy, and beta-blockers should therefore be continued indefinitely.

On the basis of these trial data, all patients should be considered for long-term oral beta-blocker after STEMI. Contraindications to beta-blocker therapy are present in around 15 per cent of patients, and consist of:

- resting heart rate <55 bpm
- second or third degree heart block
- a history of asthma.

In should be remembered that many patients with COPD have fixed obstructive defects and beta-blockers should not be excluded from all patients labelled with COPD. Since side effects and compliance can be problematic in some patients, cardioselective agents such as bisoprolol or metoprolol are preferable. Where there is concern as to whether a patient will tolerate a beta-blocker, a low dose of a short-acting prepartion can be used such as with metoprolol 25 mg bd as opposed to the usual dose of 50 mg bd. Treatment should be started on presentation for NSTEACS and once haemodynamically stable after STEMI. The dose of beta-blockers should be increased as necessary to obtain a resting heart rate of 50–60 bpm and continued indefinitely in STEMI patients.

Calcium channel blockers

Calcium channel blocking drugs have anti-ischaemic, vasodilating and antihypertensive properties that may be beneficial in patients with acute MI. A meta-analysis of more than 20 000 patients enrolled in placebo-controlled randomized trials, however, showed no significant beneficial effect on mortality. There is some evidence that the type of calcium antagonist used may be important. Dihydropyridine calcium antagonists are powerful vasodilators and may induce tachycardia, since they have no effect on the cardiac conduction system. In almost 10 000 studied patients dihydropyridine agents showed a trend towards increased mortality. Both diltiazem and verapamil have effects on the cardiac conduction system, slowing heart rate, potentially improving their efficacy in MI patients. In a series of trials randomizing 9000 patients (DAVIT-1, DAVIT-2, MDPIT and INTERCEPT), these drugs also had no significant beneficial effect on mortality, although the incidence of reinfarction and recurrent ischaemia was reduced. Subgroup analysis suggested that the overall neutral effect reflects an increase in mortality in patients with ventricular dysfunction, and a reduction in mortality in those with well-preserved ventricular function.

These studies suggest that dihydropyridine calcium antagonists should be avoided in MI patients. Rate-slowing calcium antagonists such as verapamil and diltiazem should not be given to patients with significant left ventricular dysfunction. For patients in whom a beta-blocker is contraindicated or poorly tolerated, and left ventricular function is well preserved, a rate-slowing calcium antagonist can be safely used for symptom control if required.

ACE inhibitors

Activation of the renin–angiotensin system is an early compensatory response to an evolving MI. Activation of the renin–angiotensin system leads to vasoconstriction, increased heart rate and sympathetic activation. In the early phases of evolving MI these deleterious changes will increase ventricular wall stress, increase oxygen consumption and reduce electrical stability. In the longer term, persistent activation of the renin–angiotensin system potentiates adverse remodelling, leading to ventricular dilatation and heart failure. The adverse consequences of renin–angiotensin activation can be blocked by the use of ACE inhibitors with potentially beneficial effects on mortality. More than 100 000 patients have been evaluated in a series of trials that reported in the 1990s (GISSI-3, ISIS-4, AIRE, SAVE, CCS-1 and TRACE). Trials of short-term non-selective ACE inhibitor therapy started early after MI demonstrated a small (approximately 6.5 per cent) reduction in 30-day mortality with treatment. Trials of long-term selective therapy in high-risk patients (with clinical evidence of heart failure or evidence of substantial left ventricular dysfunction) demonstrated a large (approximately 20 per cent) reduction in mortality, with particular benefit in diabetics (HOPE study). Both the HOPE and EUROPA study also showed benefit in patients with coronary disease irrespective of left ventricular function, thereby implying an additional antiatherogenic effect. On the basis of these trial data, ACE inhibitors should be prescribed early after ACS in patients who are clinically stable with an adequate blood pressure. If possible, treatment should be initiated within 24 hours of admission, titrated up to target doses. Current ACE inhibitors licensed post-MI are ramipril (target dose 5 mg bd or 10 mg od) and perindopril (target dose 8 mg od). Renal function and electrolytes should be monitored to ensure there is no significant ACE inhibitor-induced deterioration in renal function (a 20 per cent reduction in eGFR on and ACE inhibitor is acceptable). In patients who are intolerant to ACE inhibitors, angiotensin-2 receptor blocker may be used instead.

Statins

Statin therapy has been evaluated in a series of large primary and secondary prevention trials enrolling more than 50 000 patients (CARE, 4S, WOSCOPS, AFCAPS, LIPID and most recently the Heart Protection Study). These trials conclusively demonstrate that:

- statin therapy reduces mortality in patients with symptomatic ischaemic heart disease by around a third
- statin therapy is safe and well tolerated
- patients of all ages and either sex benefit

- patients with relatively normal cholesterol levels obtain similar benefit to those with substantial cholesterol elevation
- initiation of treatment in hospital helps to reduce the rate of early recurrent ischaemia and readmission.

Overall, the benefit of statin therapy in the primary prevention of coronary heart disease and in the secondary prevention of further events in patients with angina, and previous unstable angina or infarction is well-established. There is also evidence to support their role as adjunctive therapy in ACS. The rationale for this is based on their pleiotropic effects such as a positive effect on endothelial function, a reduction in platelet aggregability and an anti-inflammatory effect, manifest as a reduction in the C-reactive protein level. The MIRACL trial recruited 3000 patients with NSTEACS who were randomized to either atorvastatin 80 mg or placebo within 63 hours of presentation, in addition to routine anti-ischaemic therapy. At 4-month follow-up, there was a significant reduction in the composite end point of death/MI/resuscitated cardiac arrest/re-hospitalization for worsening angina in the treatment group, from 17.4 per cent to 14.8 per cent (p = 0.048). In addition, re-hospitalization alone was reduced as a secondary outcome. The PROVE-IT trial compared pravastatin 40 mg to atorvastatin 80 mg in both NSTEACS and STEMI. It showed a 16 per cent reduction in events (death, MI, unstable angina requiring re-hospitalization, revascularization or stroke) in those taking atorvastatin at 30 days. On the basis of these trial data, all patients with ACS should be commenced on a high dose of statin early in their hospital admission.

Hypokalaemia

Hypokalaemia is common in patients with acute infarction, and is related to prior treatment with diuretics or catecholamine effects on electrolyte handling. Hypokalaemia is associated with myocardial electrical instability (the incidence of ventricular fibrillation may be as high as 15 per cent in infarcts associated with a serum potassium of 3.0–3.5 mmol/L, and 5 per cent or less in infarcts associated with a potassium of 4.5–5.0 mmol/L) and should be corrected. If serum potassium is below 4.0 mmol/L in the absence of an important arrhythmia, then oral potassium supplements are given (e.g. slow K, three tablets three times daily, providing approximately 72 mmol potassium daily) and potassium rechecked after 12–18 hours. If ventricular arrhythmias occur in association with a serum potassium of less than 4.0 mmol/L, intravenous potassium is given as detailed in Appendix A, rechecking serum levels after 3 hours to ensure that potassium levels have risen to greater than 4.0 mmol/L.

Magnesium therapy

A number of small studies (including LIMIT-2) suggested that routine administration of magnesium may reduce mortality following acute infarction by beneficial effects on heart rate, contractility, electrical stability and platelet activity. The routine use of magnesium was therefore examined in almost 60 000 patients in the ISIS-4 study, and this showed that treatment had no beneficial effect on mortality. Subgroup analysis showed no benefit even when magnesium was given early, or to patients who did not receive thrombolytic therapy. These results were confirmed in the recent MAGIC trial of over 6000 patients. There is therefore no good evidence to support the routine use of magnesium in patients with evolving acute MI. Magnesium is, however, still indicated for the treatment of arrhythmias.

Nitrate therapy

Nitrates have a number of potentially beneficial effects (systemic vasodilatation and coronary artery dilatation), and small early studies suggested that their routine administration to patients with acute infarction may reduce mortality. The ISIS-4 and GISSI-3 trials investigated routine nitrate use in a total of almost 80 000 patients, and found no substantial beneficial effect on mortality. Although nitrates are safe and effective in the treatment of post-infarction ischaemia or heart failure, they should not routinely be administered to uncomplicated patients.

Hyperglycaemia

Patients with pre-existing diabetes have an increased risk of ischaemic heart disease, and an unfavourable prognosis following acute MI. Patients who have no history of diabetes but an elevated glucose on admission also have a poor prognosis. The high mortality may be related to the occurrence of autonomic neuropathy, pre-existing ventricular dysfunction or due to detrimental myocardial cellular changes induced by diabetes. Additionally, sympathetic activation will induce insulin resistance and hyperglycaemia in susceptible patients, increasing the release of non-esterified fatty acids, which augment myocardial oxygen consumption, depress contractility and increase the risk of heart failure. A strategy of controlling elevated plasma glucose by insulin infusion followed by subcutaneous injections in hyperglycaemic patients with acute MI could prevent these adverse metabolic effects, and was investigated in over 600 patients randomized in the DIGAMI trial. Treatment with IV insulin infusion reduced mortality by around 40 per cent. The maximum reduction in mortality occurred in patients who had not previously received insulin therapy, and were at low risk of death on the basis of clinical criteria. On the basis of these trial data, it is recommended that all patients with an admission glucose >11 mmol/L should be commenced on a sliding scale IV insulin infusion with the infusion rate adjusted to maintain blood glucose in the range 7–11 mmol/L, in combination with 500 mL of 5 per cent dextrose infused over 24 hours. Oral hypoglycaemic agents should be withdrawn. The infusion should be continued for at least 24 hours, or until the patient is clinically stable. However, it is less clear how to manage patients in the long term. The DIGAMI trial suggested that 3 months of tight glycaemic control with subcutaneous insulin may improve outcomes; however, this was not confirmed in the DIGAMI-2 trial. Therefore, tight control with conventional oral hypoglycaemics may be of benefit where possible, and may reduce the incidence of adverse effects due to insulin such as weight gain and hypoglycaemia.

Prophylactic antiarrhythmic therapy
Ventricular tachyarrhythmias are an important cause of death early after the onset of MI. Class I antiarrhythmic drugs can suppress these arrhythmias, but this beneficial effect may be offset by adverse effects such as the induction of bradyarrhythmias, induction of tachyarrhythmias and depression of ventricular function. A meta-analysis of more than 200 000 patients treated with prophylactic class I drugs showed no beneficial effects on mortality. On the basis of these trial data, routine prophylactic therapy with class I antiarrhythmic drugs early in the course of evolving MI is not recommended.

Pre-existing drug therapy
Patients admitted with evolving acute MI are often already on treatment with oral beta-blockers for pre-existing angina or hypertension. Given the beneficial effects of beta-blockers following infarction and the potential adverse effects associated with abrupt beta-blocker withdrawal, administration of these agents should continue uninterrupted unless important heart failure or a symptomatic bradyarrhythmia develops. Combined oral contraceptives and HRT are associated with an increased risk of thromboembolism and reinfarction, and should be withdrawn. Non-steroidal anti-inflammatories not only increase the risk of bleeding from the GI tract but also reduce the effectiveness of aspirin and are associated with higher rate of myocardial infarction and death. Similarly, COX-2 inhibitors should be avoided in the post-infarct period.

COMPLICATIONS OF ACS

Background

Complications following ACS are more common following STEMI. Modern reperfusion including the increased use of PCI has resulted in dramatic reductions of reinfarction and death over the last decade; consequently, this has resulted in a reduction in the incidence of post-ACS complications. In a SWISS registry of STEMI patients, reinfarction decreased from 3.7 per cent to 0.9 per cent between the years 2000 and 2007. This was linked with an increase in the use of PCI from 43 per cent to 85 per cent over the same time period. However, complications still occur and when they do arise are often related to more extensive STEMI, where the infarct-related artery has not been reperfused. This is more common in patients who present late, the elderly (over 75) and those with diabetes. These patients often have poorer left ventricular function and additionally may have extensive coronary disease which is not easily amenable to revascularization. Left ventricular dysfunction is directly associated with lower rates of survival and those with extensive myocardial injury more commonly have mechanical and arrythmic complications. In patients with severe left ventricular dysfunction (EF <30 per cent) despite successful revascularization for STEMI, the presence of pathological Q waves on ECG and signs of heart failure are clinical markers of poor myocardial recovery and prognosis. It is important to identify these patients early so they can be monitored closely and to allow for prompt treatment when necessary.

Left ventricular failure

Background

Left ventricular failure (LVF) is common after STEMI. In patients with only a small area of infarction, catecholamine-mediated increase in heart rate and contractility in the normally functioning non-infarcted segments of the left ventricle will prevent decompensation. In patients with more extensive infarction, those mechanisms are overwhelmed, left ventricular end diastolic pressure rises and pulmonary oedema occurs. In some patients, LVF is due to, or exacerbated by, complications such as arrhythmia, severe mitral regurgitation or ventricular septal rupture. The occurrence of LVF is an adverse prognostic feature, with a close correlation between the degree of failure and mortality (with in-hospital mortality rising from 6 per cent in patients free of signs of LVF, to 38 per cent in those with extensive crepitations).

Diagnosis and assessment

Clinical diagnosis of LVF after ACS is often difficult. Clinical signs, symptoms and investigational features are highly variable, inconsistent and only loosely correlated together. For example, basal crepitations are common in patients with lung disease, irrespective of the presence of LVF, and pronounced radiological pulmonary congestion can be present in a patient whose chest is clear to auscultation. LVF should be suspected in any patient with ACS and extensive ventricular dysfunction (due to a large degree of infarction, or a smaller infarction occurring in a patient with previous ischaemic ventricular damage) who develops breathlessness in association with a third heart sound and crepitations. Physical signs can change rapidly, and the heart and lungs should be auscultated at regular intervals during the early phase of evolving MI. The chest x-ray may show abnormalities including cardiomegaly, upper lobe diversion and perihilar alveolar shadowing. If signs of LVF develop, a careful clinical assessment is required (including echocardiography if possible) to exclude a mechanical complication, such as severe acute mitral regurgitation or ventricular septal rupture.

Treatment

Treatment of LVF consists of measures to relieve distress, reduce cardiac filling pressures (by vasodilatation) and decrease intraventricular fluid volume (by induction of diuresis), leading to a fall in left ventricular end diastolic pressure with resolution of pulmonary oedema. Chronic drug therapy aims to prevent the recurrence of symptoms and can reduce mortality in the case of eplerenone. This aldosterone antagonist has been shown to reduce mortality in patients with signs of post-MI heart failure and left ventricular ejection fraction of ≤ 40 per cent. This may be due to beneficial effects on reducing myocardial fibrosis or by reducing the incidence of hypokalaemia that may be an important contributing factor to fatal arrhythmias. In addition, in some patients left ventricular function will improve with resolution of myocardial stunning, helping to prevent recurrence of symptoms after the acute event. Treatment of acute LVF consists of:

- sitting the patient in an upright posture and giving oxygen. This helps to diminish venous return and improve oxygenation

- giving diamorphine by slow IV injection in 2.0 mg boluses, along with an antiemetic such as metoclopramide 10 mg. Diamorphine acts as a sedative to relieve distress, and as a vasodilator to improve pulmonary oedema

- giving a loop diuretic such as frusemide 80–160 mg as a slow intravenous injection. Intravenous loop diuretics induce vasodilatation followed by diuresis, improving LVF by a dual mechanism of action

- if blood pressure is adequate (>100 mmHg), commencing an IV nitrate infusion as detailed in Appendix A. Nitrate-induced vasodilatation helps to reduce venous return, leading to a fall in left ventricular end diastolic pressure and an improvement in pulmonary oedema. The nitrate infusion should commence at a low dose and be increased periodically

- monitor urine output accurately to ensure adequate renal perfusion and to assess response to diuretics.

If these measures fail to control the situation, a further IV bolus of frusemide should be given and a senior colleague consulted. If a surgically treatable infarct-related complication can be identified, such as acute severe mitral regurgitation or ventricular septal rupture, insertion of an intra-aortic balloon pump or assisted ventilation (which can be instituted non-invasively using mask-based systems) may help to stabilize the patient for long enough to allow corrective surgery. In the absence of a treatable complication, the prognosis of severe LVF that does not respond to diamorphine, diuretics and nitrates is poor.

Cardiogenic shock
Background
Cardiogenic shock occurs in a small proportion of patients who present with extensive infarction and is responsible for the majority of in-hospital deaths. The GRACE registry data and a large Swiss registry have shown that the incidence has recently decreased as the use of reperfusion and in particular primary PCI has increased. This is likely to be as a result of reducing recurrent ischaemia with use of stents and antiplatelets, in addition to smaller infarct sizes due to accessibility of early primary PCI and thrombolysis. Cardiogenic shock complicating an ACS can be due to:

- infarction or ischaemia of >40 per cent of the left ventricular myocardium leading to pump failure (85 per cent of cases)
- a potentially reversible complication leading to severe decompensation, such as acute mitral regurgitation, ventricular septal rupture or right ventricular infarction (15 per cent of cases).

The factors associated with an increased risk of developing cardiogenic shock are:

- extensive Q-wave anterior MI, STEMI associated with left bundle branch block or failure of reperfusion
- MI occurring in patients with previous infarction or CABG
- increasing age or female sex
- hypertension
- diabetes.

In patients who present with an extensive infarction, cardiogenic shock usually develops early (within 24 hours of admission). If cardiogenic shock develops later, a careful assessment of the patient is required. In this situation cardiogenic shock is often associated with recurrent ischaemia leading to infarct extension and further impairment of left ventricular function, or to a mechanical complication, which may be amenable to surgical correction. Data from registry studies of cardiogenic shock treated by medical therapy suggest that mortality remains around 80–90 per cent. Treatment in cardiogenic shock is designed to improve myocardial perfusion by the use of intra-aortic balloon counterpulsation and emergency revascularization. Data derived from case series, registry studies and retrospective analysis of thrombolysis trial databases suggest that early aggressive supportive therapy combined with cardiac catheterization and revascularization may favourably influence mortality. Stabilization and revascularization may be beneficial by aiding recovery of stunned myocardium around the edge of the infarct zone, allowing some recovery and improvement in myocardial function. These studies are compromised by their non-randomized trial design, and the potential confounding effect of patient selection bias, which may skew the results in favour of revascularization (since the fittest youngest patients who are most likely to survive are the cases most likely to undergo intensive treatment and revascularization). Randomized trials have been difficult to organize, but some information is now available. The Swiss Multicentre trial of Angioplasty for Shock (SMASH) demonstrated that revascularization was associated with a non-significant trend to reduced mortality although the small size of the study (55 patients) did not allow a statistically reliable conclusion to be reached. The SHould we emergently revascularize Occluded Coronaries for shocK (SHOCK) trial randomized 302 patients to receive either early revascularization or medical therapy. Survival was non-significantly improved at 30 days, and significantly improved at 6 months (50.3 per cent mortality in the revascularization group compared with 63.1 per cent mortality with medical therapy).

Subgroup analysis suggested a larger benefit for younger (<75 years of age) patients treated early (within 6 hours of diagnosis). Taken together, this body of non-randomized and randomized trial data suggests that selected patients with cardiogenic shock may benefit from intensive supportive therapy combined with revascularization.

Diagnosis

A diagnosis of cardiogenic shock due to left ventricular dysfunction can be confidently made in patients with evidence of extensive ischaemic myocardial damage who present within 24 hours of the onset of an acute STEMI with features of:

- hypotension (systolic BP persistently <90 mmHg)
- clinical signs of a low output sate (urine output <30 mL/h, poor peripheral perfusion or impaired cerebration)
- evidence of raised cardiac filling pressures (the presence of clinical or radiological pulmonary oedema implies that pulmonary artery wedge pressure is >15 mmHg).

If there are atypical features to the clinical presentation, careful evaluation is required to exclude treatable complications of MI. In particular, if there is:

- late onset of cardiogenic shock or an associated new murmur, the cardiogenic shock may be due to a mechanical complication
- low blood pressure in the absence of pulmonary oedema in a patient with inferior or posterior infarction or a negative fluid balance, when hypotension may be due to right ventricular infarction or hypovolaemia.

If any doubt exists as to the cause of the cardiogenic shock, echocardiography and pulmonary artery catheterization are required. In patients with cardiogenic shock due to severe left ventricular dysfunction there will be extensive left ventricular hypokinesia at echocardiography in association with a raised (>15 mmHg) pulmonary wedge pressure and a low (<2.2 L/min/m^2) cardiac index.

Management of cardiogenic shock due to severe ischaemic left ventricular dysfunction

In treating these patients, the priorities are to stabilize the haemodynamic situation, and identify patients who are likely to benefit from aggressive intervention. Stabilizing the haemodynamic state requires:

- treatment of arrhythmias
- giving oxygen for hypoxia

- treating pulmonary oedema with intravenous frusemide
- early percutaneous revascularization with use of intra-aortic balloon pump.

In a patient less than 75 years of age who has presented early after an infarct, cardiac catheterization and (if possible) angioplasty should be considered. Patients unsuitable for revascularization, especially those with significant co-morbidity including pre-exisiting renal impairment have a very poor prognosis and are not likely to survive. If an underlying mechanical complication such as ventricular septal rupture or acute severe mitral regurgitation is present, and surgical correction is possible, insertion of an intra-aortic balloon pump or ventilation should be considered to help stabilize the patient.

Management of hypotension associated with right ventricular infarction or hypovolaemia

Right ventricular infarction commonly occurs in association with an extensive infero-posterior STEMI due to proximal occlusion of a large right coronary artery. Ischaemic damage leads to a rise in right ventricular end diastolic pressure and reduction in right ventricular stroke volume. The infarcted dilated right ventricle impairs left ventricular filling. These two mechanisms lead to a fall in cardiac output and systemic hypotension. AF and complete heart block occur in about a third of patients with right ventricular infarction. These arrhythmias cause further haemodynamic deterioration due to loss of atrial transport in a situation where ventricular filling is already compromised. Right ventricular infarction should be suspected in any patient with inferior STEMI who develops hypotension. The diagnosis can be confirmed by:

- the presence of hypotension in association with a raised jugular venous pressure (JVP) and clear lung fields
- ST elevation in a V4R lead
- insertion of a pulmonary artery catheter and echocardiography.

Patients with right ventricular infarction as the cause of their hypotension have a characteristic haemodynamic profile, with a low or normal wedge pressure in association with a raised right ventricular diastolic and right atrial pressure. Echocardiography is required to ensure that the hypotension is not due to a ventricular septal rupture or acute severe mitral regurgitation.

Improving outcome in patients with right ventricular infarction depends on increasing right ventricular preload by fluid loading and avoiding vasodilator drugs, correcting arrhythmias and using inotropes only when fluid balance has been optimized. Treatment therefore consists of:

- insertion of a pulmonary artery catheter to confirm diagnosis and guide treatment

- avoiding treatment with diuretics or vasodilators, which will exacerbate the haemodynamic problem by reducing preload

- fluid loading with 200 mL of physiological saline over 10 minutes, followed by 1–2 litres over 2–4 hours, followed by 200 mL/h. The infusion rate should be carefully titrated to maintain an optimal wedge pressure of 15 mmHg

- if hypotension persists despite an optimal wedge pressure, treating with intravenous inotropes

- if complete heart block occurs, restoring AV synchrony with temporary dual chamber pacing

- if AF occurs, restoring AV synchrony with cardioversion.

With aggressive treatment, mortality in hypotensive patients with right ventricular infarction can be reduced to 20–30 per cent.

If fluid intake is poor or aggressive diuretic therapy has been employed, hypotension can occur in the absence of major left or right ventricular dysfunction due to intravascular volume depletion. These patients will have hypotension, clear lung fields and a normal venous pressure. A V4R recording will normally show no ST elevation. It can be difficult to confidently differentiate this from right ventricular infarction, and a pulmonary artery catheter will be required to clarify the diagnosis and guide therapy. In patients with intravascular volume depletion, wedge pressure, right ventricular and right atrial pressures will be low. Treatment consists of withholding diuretics and vasodilators and expanding intravascular volume with intravenous fluids.

Ventricular free wall rupture

Rupture of the free wall of the left ventricle occurs in up to 3 per cent of all hospitalized patients with STEMI, accounting for 20 per cent of hospital deaths. Risk factors for free wall rupture are:

- increasing age
- female sex
- first infarct

- hypertension
- marked/persistent ST elevation.

In addition, the incidence of free wall rupture may be increased by thrombolytic therapy, particularly if it is given late in the course of the infarct. Intravenous beta-blocker therapy reduces the risk of free wall rupture. Free wall ruptures present within a few days of the onset of STEMI. The usual presentation is with a sudden acute rupture presenting as collapse with electromechanical dissociation which does not respond to resuscitation. In 25 per cent of cases a subacute rupture occurs, with a slower leak of blood into the pericardial space which may produce tamponade.

Echocardiography confirms the presence of fluid in the pericardial space. Immediate surgery should be considered, as there is a high risk of major rupture and death occurring unpredictably.

Ventricular septal rupture

Ventricular septal rupture occurs in up to 2 per cent of hospitalized patients with STEMI, with most cases occurring within the first post-infarct week. With anterior infarction, the defect is usually apical and involves one direct perforation. With inferior infarction, the defect is often a complex serpiginous or fenestrated lesion involving the posterior or basal septum; these complex defects are more technically difficult to surgically repair. Patients present with signs and symptoms of heart failure in association with a new pansystolic murmur, maximal at the lower left sternal edge. The clinical presentation may be confusing, with progression to cardiogenic shock and a minimal murmur. The diagnosis can be confirmed by echocardiography or right heart catheterization. The diagnostic features are:

- visible defect in intraventricular septum with jet crossing from left to right ventricle on echocardiography

- an increase in oxygen saturation from right atrium to right ventricle of >10 per cent due to oxygenated blood crossing the septum via the defect. A large increase in saturation implies the presence of a large defect.

When the diagnosis has been established, supportive therapy with diuretics, nitrates, inotropes and an intra-aortic balloon pump may help to stabilize the haemodynamic status. Without corrective surgery, 90 per cent of patients die, usually within days of diagnosis. Even with surgery, mortality is 25–50 per cent (with mortality risk increased in older patients, those with major haemodynamic compromise, and when the defect complicates inferior infarction). Surgery should probably be carried out as early as possible, since most patients will develop progressive haemodynamic compromise with multi-organ failure if the operation is delayed, and this decreases the chance of surviving an operation. Percutaneous closure, of post-MI VSDs, with occluder devices has been successfully carried out. This is not recommended at present for routine use and patients require careful selection with regards to the position of the defect.

Acute mitral regurgitation

A mild degree of mitral regurgitation occurs in 40 per cent of patients with STEMI. This mild regurgitation is related to ventricular dilatation and shape change (which distort mitral annulus geometry) or papillary muscle dysfunction (which interferes with mitral leaflet function). The postero-medial papillary muscle is more vulnerable to ischaemia since its blood supply is derived solely from the circumflex artery, whereas the antero-lateral papillary muscle has a dual vascular supply (from the circumflex and left anterior descending). This mild degree of mitral regurgitation is usually well tolerated, and detectable only by the presence of a mitral pansystolic murmur. The mitral regurgitant murmur may be transitory, disappearing as reperfusion or recovery of left ventricular function restores mitral annulus geometry or papillary muscle function.

Severe acute mitral regurgitation complicates around 1 per cent of patients with STEMI, usually early in the first post-infarct week. The mechanism is usually rupture of the postero-medial papillary muscle complicating an inferior STEMI, leading to a flail posterior mitral leaflet. Severe acute mitral regurgitation can occur as a consequence of a small localized subendocardial infarct in a patient with well-preserved left ventricular function if the area of infarction involves the postero-medial papillary muscle. Patients present with severe heart failure, which may progress to cardiogenic shock. There may be a new loud pansystolic murmur, maximal at the apex and radiating to the axilla. If the pressure gradient between the left ventricle and left atrium is minimal (due to pressure equalization between the two chambers when the regurgitation is severe), the murmur may be minimal or absent. Even in the absence of a characteristic murmur, acute severe mitral regurgitation should be looked for in any patient who develops severe heart failure, particularly if the onset is delayed or the deterioration occurs in a patient with inferior infarction with preserved left ventricular function.

Patients with suspected acute severe mitral regurgitation require urgent evaluation with a view to emergency surgery. The diagnosis can be confirmed by:

- echocardiography; this may show a flail leaflet and Doppler evidence of severe mitral regurgitation. The left atrium is often not enlarged
- right heart catheterization and oximetry; oximetry shows no shunt, and prominent V waves may be visible in the pulmonary artery wedge pressure trace.

Treatment with diuretics, vasodilators and an intra-aortic balloon pump may help to stabilize the patient initially, but mortality without operation is >90 per cent. Urgent mitral valve surgery is required for all suitable patients. Perioperative mortality is 30 per cent and patients who survive to discharge have a good long-term prognosis.

Left ventricular thrombus, aneurysm formation and thromboembolism

The incidence of left ventricular thrombus (LVT) detected on echocardiography post-MI is around 5 per cent in the modern, reperfusion era. It is associated with poor left ventricular function and mitral regurgitation. Patients with a small degree of infarction, particularly if the site is inferior or lateral, are at lower risk. All patients with extensive anterior MI should have an early echocardiogram. If a thrombus is visualized (particularly if it is large, irregularly shaped or has frond-like appendages), there is a substantially increased risk of an early systemic embolus often leading to stroke. From observational studies, anticoagulation with warfarin has been shown to reduce the incidence of cerebral emboli in patients with LVT. However, the duration of anticoagulation has not been well established and the use of DAPT has not been investigated. Many patients require DAPT following ACS and the addition of warfarin has been shown to significantly increase the risk of major bleeding. Therefore warfarin and DAPT should only be used in patients with LVT at highest risk of thromboembolism such as those with AF and poor left ventricular function. Ideally the treatment should be switched to warfarin alone or with a single antiplatelet agent as soon as reasonably possible, which usually depends on the type of stent used at revascularization.

Left ventricular aneurysm (LVA) develops in a large proportion of patients with complicated extensive infarcts and is often associated with LVT and heart failure. The clinical features that increase the risk of LVA formation are:

- extensive anterior STEMI
- persistent ST elevation in the infarct zone
- heart failure.

Patients with confirmed LVA should be considered for anticoagulation to reduce thromboembolism. In view of their concomitant left ventricular dysfunction they should also receive adequate drug therapy, including ACE inhibitors and aldosterone antagonists. They are at high risk of ventricular arrhythmia and should be evaluated for an implantable cardioverter defibrillator (ICD). If they remain symptomatic with heart failure or develop worsening mitral regurgitation, due to negative left ventricular remodelling, they should be considered for coronary artery bypass surgery and aneurysmectomy.

Clinically significant deep venous thrombosis and pulmonary embolism are now rare following uncomplicated ACS. The risks are increased in patients with extensive complicated STEMI, particularly if prolonged bed rest or heart failure occur. In high-risk patients, prophylactic low-dose subcutaneous LMWH should be instituted and continued until the patient is clinically stable and mobile.

Pericarditis

Pericarditis is an early complication associated with extensive STEMI, usually within the first week. The clinical features of pericarditis complicating anterior STEMI are:

- sharp central chest pain, worse with respiration, relieved by sitting up or leaning forward but not relieved by glyceryl trinitrate (GTN)
- an associated friction rub.

In inferior STEMI a friction rub is rare, and the pain may be atypical or radiate to the left shoulder. Progression of pericarditis to a clinically significant effusion is rare. Treatment consists of:

- reassuring the patient about the cause of the symptoms
- pain relief with simple analgesics such as dihydrocodeine, with non-steroidal anti-inflammatory agents reserved for patients with persistent symptoms
- avoiding administration of anticoagulants if possible, as they may increase the risk of progression to haemorrhagic pericardial effusion, leading to tamponade.

Patients who present later (between 2 weeks and 3 months post-MI) with pericardial pain and friction rub, fever and an elevated erythrocyte sedimentation rate (ESR) may have Dressler's syndrome. This is thought to be an immunological syndrome triggered by myocardial necrosis. Patients may have associated pleurisy and, rarely, pulmonary infiltrates. Dressler's syndrome is now rare after MI, and is seen most commonly after cardiac surgery.

EARLY PERI-INFARCTION ARRHYTHMIAS

Background

Peri-infarction arrhythmias (occurring within 48 hours) are very common in patients with STEMI, and are an important cause of death. Acute myocardial ischaemia induces a wide range of detrimental changes in myocyte metabolism (intracellular acidosis, raised cAMP, raised sodium, magnesium and calcium). These occur in association with adverse changes in systemic biochemical and physiological function induced by the evolving infarct (systemic acidosis, abnormal potassium, lactate, adenosine, CO_2 and lysophosphoglycerides along with catecholamine release and autonomic disturbance). These factors interact to destabilize myocardial electrical function, leading to the induction of peri-infarction arrhythmias. Even a small area of ischaemia or infarction can develop electrical instability, leading to the induction of potentially lethal arrhythmias. These local and systemic proarrhythmic disturbances are maximal early after the onset of the ACS, resolving within 48 hours, thereby reducing the risk of late arrhythmia recurrence due to these mechanisms. Since these early peri-infarction arrhythmias are not related to infarct size and have a low recurrence rate, they are not invariably associated with a poor long-term prognosis.

Infarct site has an important influence on the type of peri-infarction arrhythmias that occur. In patients with anterior infarction there is a relative excess of sympathetic activation, promoting the induction of tachyarrhythmias in areas of enhanced automaticity. There is a high density of vagal receptors in the infero-posterior wall of the left ventricle, which are activated during inferior infarction. The resultant increase in vagal activity, acting in conjunction with infarct-related disturbance of function in the conduction system, increases the incidence of bradyarrhythmias.

Supraventricular and ventricular ectopic beats

Frequent ectopic beats occur in the majority of patients with ACS. Supraventricular ectopic beats are due to enhanced automaticity in the atria or AV junction. Since ventricular activation occurs via the normal conduction system, supraventricular ectopics are characterized by a QRS complex of normal morphology, which occurs prematurely and may be preceded by an abnormal P wave. Ventricular ectopics arise due to enhanced automaticity in the ventricular myocardium. Since depolarization occurs outside the normal conduction system, the resultant QRS complex has a broad configuration. Ectopic beats are usually asymptomatic, and are not associated with an adverse prognosis, regardless of their frequency and complexity. When frequent ectopics occur:

- pain relief should be adequate – if continuing ischaemic pain is present, use of IV beta-blockade or further diamorphine should be considered
- heart failure should be looked for and treated if present
- electrolytes should be checked and oral supplements given if potassium is <4.0 mmol/L
- giving IV magnesium should be considered if the patient has been on long-term diuretic therapy prior to admission.

There is no evidence that suppression of ectopics with antiarrhythmic drugs prevents the occurrence of life-threatening arrhythmias or improves prognosis.

Sinus tachycardia

Sinus tachycardia is common after an ACS, and is often associated with extensive anterior STEMI, sympathetic activation and an adverse prognosis. In sinus tachycardia, each QRS complex is preceded by a normal P wave, the QRS complexes are of normal morphology, and the rate is normally less than 140 bpm. If sinus tachycardia is persistent and excessive, it may cause extension of myocardial necrosis by increasing oxygen consumption. If sinus tachycardia is persistent:

- adequate analgesia should be ensured
- heart failure should be looked for and treated
- beta-blockade should be considered if there are no contraindications.

Prolonged sinus tachycardia is most likely to occur in a patient with extensive infarction and major left ventricular impairment.

Atrial tachyarrhythmias

Peri-infarction AF occurs in 10–20 per cent of STEMI patients. Atrial electrical instability or stretch leads to the development of multiple micro re-entry circuits within the atrium leading to chaotic atrial electrical activity which is intermittently conducted via the AV node to erratically depolarize the ventricles. The rapid ventricular rate and loss of AV synchrony results in a significant reduction in cardiac output and an increase in ischaemia. Characteristic ECG features of AF are an irregular baseline due to fibrillation waves (often best seen in V1) with completely irregular ventricular activity. The incidence of AF is increased in patients with:

- large infarctions
- increased age
- pericarditis
- right ventricular infarction
- diabetes
- hypertension
- inotrope use.

The development of early (<24 hours) AF is usually associated with inferior STEMI, whilst later (>24 hours) AF is usually associated with anterior STEMI and heart failure. Mortality is more than doubled in ACS patients who develop AF.

The treatment of ACS-related AF depends on the ventricular rate and associated clinical features:

- If the ventricular rate is rapid (>200 bpm), systolic BP is low (<90 mmHg) or the arrhythmia is associated with chest pain, heart failure or impaired consciousness, immediate direct current cardioversion (DCC) is the treatment of choice.

- Many episodes of ACS-related AF are short-lived (50 per cent last less than 30 minutes) and well tolerated. If AF occurs with a rate of <110 bpm, systolic blood pressure is maintained above 90 mmHg and there are no associated symptoms, no treatment is necessary initially.

- If AF persists for more than 30 minutes, has a rate consistently >110 bpm, is associated with a fall in systolic BP or with rate-related symptoms, drug treatment is indicated.

A variety of drugs can be used to treat patients with peri-infarction AF. In patients with coexistent symptomatic left ventricular dysfunction, digoxin (0.25–0.5 mg IV every 6–8 hours up to a maximum of 1 mg/24 hours) helps to slow ventricular rate and its inotropic properties may improve cardiac function. Digoxin slows ventricular rate by an indirect effect on AV nodal conduction, mediated by an increase in parasympathetic activity. In patients with acute infarction who have extensive sympathetic activation and vagal inhibition, this mechanism may be relatively ineffective. In patients who have no signs of heart failure (or other contraindication), IV atenolol is effective for rapid ventricular rate control. If a central venous line is in place, intravenous amiodarone is useful. This can be administered to patients regardless of left ventricular function. In addition to achieving rapid ventricular rate control (due to a beta-blocking effect) amiodarone also has a beneficial effect on atrial electrical stability. This helps to restore sinus rhythm in up to 75 per cent of treated patients within 4 hours.

All patients with AF should be anticoagulated with heparin. If the arrhythmia persists for more than 24 hours, restoration of sinus rhythm by electrical cardioversion should be considered to reduce the long-term risk of arrhythmia-associated thromboembolism. Atrial flutter is less common than AF, but presents and is managed in a similar fashion.

Idioventricular rhythm

Idioventricular rhythm is very common in STEMI patients, presenting as a regular broad complex tachycardia with a stable QRS configuration and a rate of less than 120 bpm. It is due to enhanced automaticity in a ventricular focus, and is often associated with spontaneous or therapeutic reperfusion. Idioventricular rhythm is rarely associated with haemodynamic compromise and has no adverse effect on mortality. Since the arrhythmia is usually well tolerated, no specific treatment is required.

Ventricular tachycardia

Non-sustained VT (three or more consecutive ventricular beats at a rate >120 bpm, lasting for less than 30 seconds) occurs in up to 7 per cent of STEMI patients. When it occurs in patients with previous MI or has a rapid rate, it may be a marker of an adverse prognosis. In most patients it is asymptomatic, and antiarrhythmic therapy (with the exception of beta-blockers) should be avoided. As for other non-sustained peri-infarction arrhythmias, treatment should be directed towards control of pain, ongoing cardiac ischaemia, heart failure and correction of electrolyte disturbance. If episodes of non-sustained VT are frequent, prolonged or symptomatic, and do not respond to the above measures or beta-blockers and magnesium then amiodarone can be considered if the corrected QT interval is normal.

Sustained VT (lasting for >30 seconds) is relatively uncommon, occurring in up to 2 per cent of STEMI patients. The occurrence of sustained VT is associated with extensive ventricular dysfunction and recurrent ischaemia, and is therefore a marker of increased hospital mortality. Monomorphic VT presents as a regular broad complex tachycardia with a rate >120 bpm. Polymorphic VT presents as a broad complex tachycardia with variable morphology. Polymorphic VT is usually rapid and poorly tolerated. Sustained VT has important adverse effects in post-infarct patients, leading to:

- hypotension and heart failure if the ventricular rate is rapid and left ventricular function poor
- ischaemia and infarct extension due to increased myocardial oxygen consumption
- further electrical instability (exacerbated by the above mechanisms) leading to VF.

The onset of sustained VT is therefore a medical emergency. Treatment selection depends on the degree of haemodynamic compromise and the underlying cause:

- If systolic BP <90 mmHg or the patient has chest pain, a reduced conscious level or heart failure related to the tachycardia, DCC is the treatment of choice. If consciousness is lost with the onset of VT, the shock should be administered immediately. If the patient remains conscious, despite haemodynamic compromise, sedation with 2–10 mg IV midazolam is given prior to cardioversion.

- Patients with ischaemic substrate for VT should be considered for intra-aortic balloon pump and revascularization if VT is refractory to other treatment.

- If systolic BP >90 mmHg and the patient is not distressed or poorly perfused, initial treatment should be with amiodarone 300 mg IV over 1 hour, followed by an infusion of 900 mg over 24 hours. If VT persists and the patient deteriorates haemodynamically during amiodarone administration, immediate DCC should be performed.

- Torsade de Pointes, where the QT interval may be prolonged, should be treated with correction of the underlying cause (i.e. drug toxicity or hypokalaemia) as well as giving IV magnesium. If refractory to treatment, then temporary pacing either via the right atrium or right ventricle should be considered with the aim of increasing the heart rate to >90bpm.

- Temporary overdrive pacing may also be effective in terminating episodes of resistant VT. A pacing lead should be inserted into the right ventricle. When VT occurs, pacing therapy should be instituted at a rate 20 per cent faster than the VT for 10 seconds, then abruptly discontinued. If the pacing therapy is successful, sinus rhythm will return. The ECG should be checked and pacing instituted if the QT interval is prolonged. Rapid VT or VF may be precipitated by overdrive pacing, requiring immediate cardioversion. The addition of high-dose beta-blockade, and haemodynamic support with a balloon pump, may also help to suppress the arrhythmia.

Since these arrhythmias are often associated with left ventricular impairment or recurrent ischaemia, treatment with diuretics, nitrates and anti-ischaemic agents should be optimized, and early cardiac catheterization considered.

Ventricular fibrillation

Ventricular fibrillation is characterized by rapid disorganized multiple re-entrant wavelets in the ventricle, resulting in loss of co-ordinated ventricular myocyte activity with loss of output and cardiac arrest. Untreated, the arrhythmia is fatal, and is responsible for most pre-hospital deaths in patients with STEMI. Most episodes occur early, with 80 per cent occurring within 12 hours of symptom onset. If defibrillation is performed rapidly, most episodes of VF can be reversed, but success rate declines rapidly with time. When VF occurs early in patients with good left ventricular function, long-term survival is not compromised; when VF occurs late in patients with heart failure, it is often a terminal event. The protocol for treatment of VF is detailed in Chapter 2.

Sinus bradycardia

Sinus bradycardia (<60 bpm) is common early after ACS, particularly in patients with inferior STEMI and vagal activation. If the heart rate is persistently below 45 bpm or there are rate-related symptoms, a bolus of atropine 0.6 mg IV (repeated as necessary) will increase the sinus rate. If sinus bradycardia persists despite repeated boluses of atropine, temporary pacing should be considered.

Conduction disturbances in relation to infarct site

A variety of conduction disturbances can occur in patients with evolving STEMI. Although early reperfusion has shortened the duration of symptomatic episodes and reduced the need for temporary pacing, the incidence of AV block has remained relatively constant. When a conduction disturbance occurs in a patient with inferior STEMI, it is usually due to vagal activation, AV nodal ischaemia, or both. If complete heart block develops, it is usually well tolerated. Since there is no damage to the conduction system in the ventricles, a secondary pacemaker in the bundle of His takes over ventricular activation, producing a stable reliable rhythm with a rate of >40 bpm, which is usually sufficient to maintain the circulation with no compromise. This escape rhythm is conducted via the normal ventricular activation pathways, and therefore will have a narrow QRS configuration. Normal AV nodal function recovers within hours or days, with a return to normal sinus rhythm.

By contrast, when AV block develops in a patient with anterior STEMI, it is often poorly tolerated and is associated with a high risk of early death. For AV block to occur in anterior STEMI, extensive and widespread damage to the left ventricular myocardium and the interventricular septum must occur, and the patients often die from heart failure. In these patients, the conduction disturbance is related to infarction of the bundle of His within the interventricular septum. The secondary pacemaker that is responsible for ventricular activation will be situated outside the specialized conduction system in the surviving ventricular myocardium. The escape rhythm generated by this type of secondary pacemaker will often have an unreliable rate of <40 bpm (since the inherent automaticity of cells outside the specialized conduction system is usually low), and will have a broad QRS configuration as ventricular activation will be slow. This slow rate will be poorly tolerated in a patient with extensive ventricular damage, and episodes of unpredictable ventricular asystole often occur. When AV block occurs following acute anterior STEMI, temporary pacing is usually required. If the patient survives the acute episode, the AV block is often persistent or recurrent, and a permanent pacemaker may be required.

In extensive anterior STEMI with involvement of the septum, ischaemic damage to the bundle of His may lead to left or right bundle branch block on the surface EGG. The development of left bundle branch block usually indicates that extensive myocardial necrosis has occurred, with associated significant left ventricular dysfunction and a poor prognosis.

Right bundle branch block can occur with less extensive infarction, as can involvement of only the anterior fascicle of the left bundle, leading to left axis deviation. Patients who develop left bundle branch block in combination with a long PR interval, or the combination of right bundle branch block, left axis deviation and a long PR interval, have suffered extensive damage to their conduction system; such patients should be discussed with a senior colleague, as prophylactic temporary pacing may be indicated to avert the need for pacemaker insertion in a compromised patient if sudden complete heart block with a slow escape rhythm develops.

First degree heart block

First degree AV block manifests with prolongation of the PR interval (Figure 1.8). It is the most common conduction disturbance, occurring in up to 15 per cent of patients, usually associated with inferior STEMI. Progression to self-terminating and well-tolerated episodes of high-grade AV block is common. No specific treatment is required, other than withholding drugs (such as beta-blockers or digoxin), which impair AV nodal conduction, and closely monitoring the patient.

Mobitz type 1 (Wenckebach) heart block

Mobitz type 1 block is common after inferior STEMI. It often occurs in patients who progress from first degree, through Mobitz type 1 to well tolerated complete block with a narrow complex escape rhythm. The ECG shows a progressive increase in PR interval culminating in a complete failure of conduction and a dropped beat. Apart from avoiding AV nodal blocking drugs, no treatment other than close observation is required.

Mobitz type 2 second degree block

Mobitz type 2 block is less common, and manifests itself as sudden unpredictable failure of AV nodal conduction, resulting in a dropped beat with no preceding change in the PR interval. Mobitz type 2 block is usually associated with septal involvement in extensive anterior STEMI, leading to ischaemic damage to the bundle of His, and often coexists with bundle branch block. Mobitz type 2 block frequently progresses to poorly tolerated complete heart block with a slow and unreliable broad complex escape rhythm. Patients with anterior STEMI who develop Mobitz type 2 block have a poor prognosis. When Mobitz type 2 block occurs, a senior colleague should be consulted, as prophylactic temporary pacing may be indicated to avert the need for pacemaker

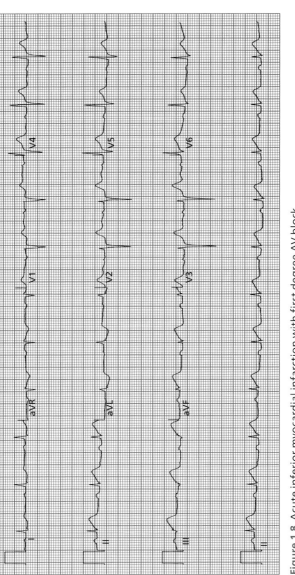

Figure 1.8 Acute inferior myocardial infarction with first degree AV block.

insertion in a compromised patient if sudden complete heart block with a slow escape rhythm develops.

Third degree (complete) heart block

Complete heart block occurs in up to 6 per cent of STEMI, and presents with complete dissociation between atrial and ventricular activity (Figure 1.9). The pathophysiology and recommended treatment depend on the site of infarction associated with the heart block.

In inferior STEMI, patients usually progress through first degree and Wenckebach block to well-tolerated complete heart block with a narrow complex escape rhythm. If the blood pressure is well maintained and the patient is asymptomatic, no treatment is necessary. If the ventricular rate falls below 40 bpm, pauses of >3 seconds occur, the systolic BP falls below 90 mmHg or rate-related symptoms develop:

- atropine 0.6 mg should be given IV, repeated as necessary
- if symptomatic complete heart block persists despite atropine, a temporary pacing wire should be inserted.

Normal AV nodal conduction usually returns within 48 hours, a permanent pacemaker is not required, and prognosis after discharge from hospital is good.

In patients with anterior STEMI, complete heart block often occurs suddenly, particularly in patients who develop left bundle branch block or have a period of Mobitz type 2 block. The escape rhythm is broad, complex and slow, often associated with severe haemodynamic compromise in a patient with extensive infarction and major left ventricular impairment. Temporary pacing is always required to maintain an adequate rate. High-grade AV block often persists, necessitating permanent pacemaker implantation. A large proportion of patients who develop complete heart block following anterior STEMI die, often from pump failure due to ventricular damage.

Permanent cardiac pacing after STEMI

In patients with inferior STEMI, high-degree AV block is usually self-limiting, but can persist for up to 2 weeks. Patients with high-degree block that persists beyond this point will require a permanent pacing system. In patients with anterior STEMI and high-degree block, even if transient, there is a high risk of subsequent asystole and a permanent pacing system implant is recommended.

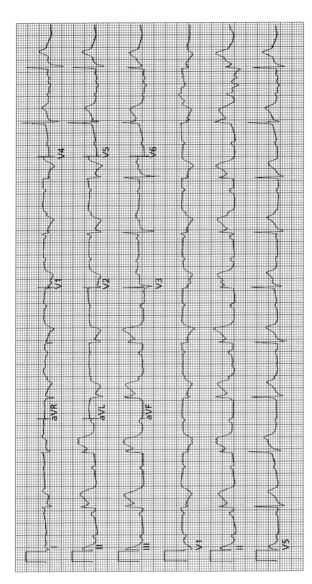

Figure 1.9 Acute inferior myocardial infarction with complete AV block.

LATE POST-INFARCTION ARRHYTHMIAS

Background

Arrhythmias that develop more than 48 hours after the onset of STEMI have a different pathophysiology and therapeutic approach. Many of the arrhythmias are related to the formation of fibrosis in the infarct zone. Myocardial fibrosis slows and disturbs conduction, resulting in the development of re-entry circuits that are electrically unstable and generate ventricular tachyarrhythmias. Since these late arrhythmias have a chronic substrate, they are likely to be recurrent. Because of this, they are a common cause of post-infarction mortality, and are a marker of a poor prognosis.

Frequent ventricular ectopic beats

The presence of frequent ventricular ectopic beats in the post-infarction period (>10/h) is strongly associated with an adverse prognosis. More than 100 000 patients have been studied in randomized trials investigating the use of class I and class III antiarrhythmic drugs to suppress ventricular ectopics in the hope of preventing subsequent malignant arrhythmias. None of the large well-conducted trials has shown a mortality benefit (and some have shown an adverse pro-arrhythmic effect). In patients with frequent ventricular ectopics, secondary preventative therapy with ACE inhibitors and beta-blockers should be optimized and revascularization performed if there is ongoing ischaemia; antiarrhythmic drug therapy should not be prescribed.

Ventricular tachycardia

Ventricular tachycardia occurring after the first 48 hours, even if asymptomatic or non-sustained, is an important risk factor for early sudden death, particularly when it occurs in association with significant left ventricular dysfunction (ejection fraction <35 per cent). Trials of class I antiarrhythmic drugs have been uniformly disappointing, with no beneficial effect, and some evidence of an adverse pro-arrhythmic effect. In the late 1990s, five important trials (EMIAT, CAMIAT, MADIT, MADIT-2 and MUST) reported, and provide some guidelines for an evidence-based approach to management of these patients. Current guidelines state that patients who have syncopal VT or VF without a treatable cause (i.e. not related to their index presentation) should be considered for an ICD for secondary prevention. Patients who are over 1 month from their index event qualify for an ICD on primary grounds if they have an ejection fraction (EF) of <30 per cent and QRS duration of ≥120 ms or if the EF is <35 per cent with non-sustained VT on holter monitor and inducible VT on electrophysiological testing. Therefore, all patients with impaired left ventricular function should be carefully evaluated to assess who will require further investigation.

RECOVERY AND REHABILITATION

The in-hospital recovery period

Following admission with ACS, all patients should remain on bed rest with continuous rhythm monitoring and close supervision in a CCU environment for at least 24 hours. This is the period of time when the risk of a potentially fatal but reversible arrhythmia is high. In addition, multiple therapeutic interventions designed to reduce infarct size, stabilize the patient and improve prognosis are required. Management after this first 24-hour period will depend on clinical stability and risk profile. Patients who have a small ACS (localized ECG changes and small enzyme rise) who are clinically stable with no complications after 24 hours generally have a good prognosis. These uncomplicated patients can begin to mobilize and undertake self-care after 24 hours, and be transferred out of the CCU to a less intensively monitored ward environment. Hospital stay should be limited to 2–3 days for uncomplicated patients who have been successfully treated by either PCI or with thrombolysis and subsequent PCI. Those that have been managed conservatively without coronary angiography should remain in hospital for 5–7 days and should be considered for other means of risk stratification if appropriate. By discharge, patients should be walking 200 metres on the level and up a flight of stairs without symptoms. The occurrence of any ischaemia, heart failure, dysrhythmia or other complications during the mobilization phase indicates the need for careful reassessment with a view to determining the need for further investigation prior to discharge.

Patients who have extensive myocardial injury (widespread ECG changes and large enzyme rise) are at increased risk of early complications, and remain unstable for a more prolonged period of time. These complicated patients need to stay on CCU for intensive treatment and monitoring, with a large proportion requiring cardiac catheterization, PCI, cardiac surgery or arrhythmia intervention prior to hospital discharge. High-risk patients who are stabilized should be transferred out of CCU with a view to discharge after slow mobilization. Patients and relatives should be provided with verbal and written information about their condition, and referred to a rehabilitation programme.

Rehabilitation

After ACS, cardiac rehabilitation aims to restore patients to their optimal physical, psychosocial, emotional and vocational status using a multidisciplinary and multifactorial programme. Each patient needs a programme tailored to meet individual needs. As a minimum, sessions of medical assessment and review, education and counselling should be offered to all patients. Patients who make a good recovery from their ACS and have a satisfactory negative exercise test should enter a supervised exercise programme. In patients with extensive infarction or a positive exercise test, exercise rehabilitation should be deferred until investigation and further treatment are completed. Patients who have important co-morbidity may not be suitable for an exercise programme. Patients who complete a multifactorial rehabilitation programme benefit from:

- reduced anxiety and depression
- increased chance of returning to active employment
- improved cardiovascular function and exercise capacity
- optimized risk factor management.

These beneficial effects combine to improve prognosis, with meta-analysis of over 2000 patients enrolled in randomized studies suggesting that rehabilitation programmes reduce readmission rates and improve mortality by about 25 per cent over 3 years.

Lifestyle modification and general advice

Smoking cessation after ACS reduces the rate of progression of coronary disease. Cardiac event rates are reduced by 50 per cent. Access to specialized smoking cessation clinics should be available for all smokers. Reducing the number of cigarettes smoked, or changing to cigars or a pipe, is not an effective way of reducing risk. Even consumption of one cigarette a day doubles the risk of further ACS. Passive smoking has a similar adverse effect as smoking one cigarette daily, and partners of ACS survivors should be encouraged to stop. A diet low in saturated fat and calories but high in carbohydrates, fruit, vegetables, fibre and fish has favourable effects on lipid profile, blood pressure and haemostatic risk factors, and is recommended after ACS. An active lifestyle with regular exercise and stress management techniques improves quality of life and may have beneficial effects on survival. Although consumption of low levels of alcohol may be cardioprotective, high levels of alcohol consumption (more than three units per day) are associated with hypertension and increased mortality, and should be discouraged.

The Driver and Vehicle Licensing Agency (DVLA) does not require that patients inform them after an uncomplicated ACS, although patients are not allowed to drive for up 4 weeks unless successfully treated with primary PCI and the EF is ≥40 per cent, in which case driving can commence after 1 week. After a complicated ACS the DVLA may impose a large period of restriction, and patients should be advised to contact the authority directly for advice. The requirements of insurance companies are variable. Patients should seek advice from their own insurer before recommencing driving after ACS. Patients who hold a vocational licence to drive an HGV or public service vehicle must contact the DVLA after an ACS. These licences will be automatically withdrawn, but may be returned if the DVLA is satisfied with a medical report and the results of a post-ACS exercise test (currently patients are required to exercise for 9 minutes of the Bruce protocol, off medical therapy, with no symptoms or ECG changes). Air travel should be avoided for 6 weeks after an uncomplicated ACS or longer in patients with complications. Sexual activity should be avoided early after ACS. Patients who have a satisfactory exercise test result can be reassured that the cardiovascular demands of intercourse are normally less than of the exercise test, and be encouraged to return to normal activity. Patients with significant post-MI exercise symptoms may need more specialized psychosexual counselling.

KEY POINTS

- ACS are very common. Although modern treatment has improved outcome in younger patients, ageing of the population results in a continuing high prevalence of morbidity and mortality.

- Most deaths occur shortly after the onset of symptoms.

- Almost all episodes of ACS are caused by thrombotic occlusion or partial occlusion of a coronary artery related to an unstable atherosclerotic lesion.

- Plaque instability (reflecting enhanced inflammatory activity within an atherosclerotic lesion) may be triggered by multiple factors.

- Initial categorization of an ACS is based on clinical evaluation combined with analysis of the ECG.

- Cardiac troponins are highly sensitive and specific biomarkers, with elevation confirming that irreversible myocardial necrosis has occurred.

- Emergency treatment requires analgesia, antiplatelet drugs, treatment of hypokalaemia and hyperglycaemia and appropriate reperfusion therapy.

- Where available, primary PCI is superior to thrombolysis.

- Beta-blockers, ACE inhibitors and statins should be instituted in all suitable patients.

- Heart failure and hypotension require careful evaluation.

- Mechanical complications are relatively rare but associated with high rates of morbidity and mortality.

- Many arrhythmias are transient and self-terminating.

- Active rehabilitation after MI improves long-term outcome.

KEY REFERENCES

ACC/AHA 2007 Guidelines for the management of patients with unstable angina/non-ST-elevation myocardial infarction – executive summary. *J Am Coll Cardiol* 2007; **50**: 652–726.

ACE Inhibition Myocardial Infarction Collaborative Group. Indications for ACE inhibitors in the early treatment of acute myocardial infarction. Systemic overview of individual data from 100000 patients in randomised trials. *Circulation* 1998; **97**: 2202–12.

Antman EM, Cohen M, Radley D, et al. Assessment of the treatment effect of enoxaparin for unstable angina/non-Q-wave myocardial infarction. TIMI 11B-ESSENCE meta-analysis. *Circulation* 1999; **100**: 1602–8.

Bavry AA, Bhatt DL, et al. Benefit of early invasive therapy in acute coronary syndromes: a meta-analysis of contemporary randomized clinical trials. *J Am Coll Cardiol* 2006; **48**: 1319–25.

Boersma E, et al. Does time matter? A pooled analysis of randomized clinical trials comparing primary percutaneous coronary intervention and in-hospital fibrinolysis in acute myocardial infarction patients. *Eur Heart J* 2006; **27**: 779–88.

Bonaca MP, et al. Antithrombotics in acute coronary syndromes. *J Am Coll Cardiol* 2009; **54**: 969–84.

Borden WB, Faxon DP. Facilitated percutaneous coronary intervention. *J Am Coll Cardiol* 2006; **48**: 1120–8.

Brodie BR, Stuckey TD. Mechanical reperfusion therapy for acute myocardial infarction: Stent PAMI, ADMIRAL, CADILLAC and beyond. *Heart* 2002; **87**: 191–2.

Brown N, Young T, Gray D, Skene AM, Hampton JR. Inpatient deaths from acute myocardial infarction, 1982–92: analysis of data in the Nottingham heart attack register. *BMJ* 1997; **315**: 159–64.

Budaj A, Yusuf S, et al. Benefit of clopidogrel in patients with acute coronary syndromes without ST-segment elevation in various risk groups. *Circulation* 2002; **106**: 1622–6.

Burzotta F, et al. Clinical impact of thrombectomy in acute ST-elevation myocardial infarction: an individual patient-data pooled analysis of 11 trials. *Eur Heart J* 2009; **30**: 2193–203.

Cantor WJ, et al. Routine early angioplasty after fibrinolysis for acute myocardial infarction. *N Engl J Med* 2009; **360**: 2705–18.

Causer JP, Connelly DT. Implantable defibrillators for life threatening ventricular arrhythmias are more effective than antiarrhythmic drugs in selected high risk patients. *BMJ* 1998; **317**: 762–3.

Channer K, Morris F. ABC of clinical electrocardiography. Myocardial ischaemia. *BMJ* 2002; **324**: 1023–6.

Chen Z, et al. Addition of clopidogrel to aspirin in 45 852 patients with acute myocardial infarction: randomised placebo-controlled trial. *Lancet* 2005; **366**: 1607–21.

Chen Z, et al. Early intravenous then oral metoprolol in 45 852 patients with acute myocardial infarction: randomised placebo- controlled trial. *Lancet* 2005; **366**: 1622–32.

Collet J, Montalescot G, et al. Percutaneous coronary intervention after fibrinolysis: a multiple meta-analyses approach according to the type of strategy. *J Am Coll Cardiol* 2006; **48**: 1326–35.

Cuisset T, et al. Benefit of a 600-mg loading dose of clopidogrel on platelet reactivity and clinical outcomes in patients with non-ST-segment elevation acute coronary syndrome undergoing coronary stenting. *J Am Coll Cardiol* 2006; **48**: 1339–45.

Davies MJ. The pathophysiology of acute coronary syndromes. *Heart* 2000; **83**: 361–6.

de Belder MA. Acute myocardial infarction: failed thromboysis. *Heart* 2001; **85**: 104–12.

De Luca G, Suryapranata H, Stone GW, et al. Abciximab as adjunctive therapy to reperfusion in acute ST-Segment elevation myocardial infarction: a meta-analysis of randomized trials. *JAMA* 2005; **293**(14): 1759–65.

De Luca G, Suryapranata H, et al. Time delay to treatment and mortality in primary angioplasty for acute myocardial infarction: every minute of delay counts. *Circulation* 2004; **109**: 1223–5.

Edhouse J, Brady WJ, Morris F. ABC of clinical electrocardiography. Acute myocardial infarction – Part II. *BMJ* 2002; **324**: 963–6.

Fernandez-Avilés F, et al. Routine invasive strategy within 24 hours of thrombolysis versus ischaemia-guided conservative approach for acute myocardial infarction with ST-segment elevation (GRACIA-1): a randomised controlled trial. *Lancet* 2004; **364**: 1045–53.

Freemantle N, Cleland J, Young P, Mason J, Harrison J. B blockade after myocardial infarction: systemic review and meta regression analysis. *BMJ* 1999; **318**: 1730–7.

Gershlick AH, et al. Rescue angioplasty after failed thrombolytic therapy for acute myocardial infarction. *N Engl J Med* 2005; **353**: 2758–68.

Ghuran A, Camm AJ. Periinfarction arrhythmias. In: Kowey PJ, Podrid PR (eds), *Cardiac Arrhythmias: Mechanisms, Diagnosis and Management*. Philadelphia: Lippincott, Williams and Wilkins, 2001.

Goncalves A, et al. TIMI, PURSUIT, and GRACE risk scores: sustained prognostic value and interaction with revascularization in NSTE-ACS. *Eur Heart J* 2005; **26**: 865–72.

Hamm CW, Goldmann BU, Heeschen C, Kreymann G, Berger J, Meinertz T. Emergency room triage of patients with acute chest pain by means of rapid testing for cardiac troponin T or troponin I. *N Engl J Med* 1997; **337**(23): 1648–53.

Hlatky MA. Evaluation of chest pain in the emergency department. *N Engl J Med* 1997; **337**(23): 1687–8.

Implantable cardioverter defibrillators for arrhythmias. Review of Technology Appraisal 11. *National Institute for Health and Clinical Excellence* January 2006.

Keeley EC, Boura JA, Grimes CL. Primary angioplasty versus intravenous thrombolytic therapy for acute myocardial infarction: a quantitative review of 23 randomised trials. *Lancet* 2003; **361**: 13–20.

Keeley EC, Boura JA, Grimes CL. Comparison of primary and facilitated percutaneous coronary interventions for ST-elevation myocardial infarction: quantitative review of randomised trials. *Lancet* 2006; **367**: 579–88.

Laarman GJ, Dirksen MT. Early discharge after primary PCI. *Heart* 2010; **96**: 584–7.

Mahon NG, O'Rorke C, Codd MB, McCann HA, McGarry K, Sugrue DD. Hospital mortality of acute myocardial infarction in the thrombolytic era. *Heart* 1999; **81**: 478–82.

Malmberg K, Ryden L, Efendic S, et al. Randomised trial of insulin-glucose infusion followed by subcutaneous insulin treatment in diabetic patients with acute myocardial infarction (DIGAMI study): effects on mortality at 1 year. *J Am Coll Cardiol* 1995; **26**: 57–65.

Mehta SR, et al. Early versus delayed invasive intervention in acute coronary syndromes. *N Engl J Med* 2009; **360**: 2165–75.

Montalescot G, Cayla G, Collet J, et al. Immediate vs delayed intervention for acute coronary syndromes: a randomized clinical trial. *JAMA* 2009; **302**(9): 947–54.

Morris F, Brady WJ. ABC of clinical electrocardiography. Acute myocardial infarction – Part I. *BMJ* 2002; **324**: 831–4.

Murphy JJ. Problems with temporary cardiac pacing. *BMJ* 2001; **323**: 527.

Nattrass M. Managing diabetes after myocardial infarction. *BMJ* 1997; **314**: 1497.

Noble MIM. Can negative results for protein markers of myocardial damage justify discharge of acute chest pain patients after a few hours in hospital? *Eur Heart J* 1999; **20**: 925–7.

Norris RM. The natural history of acute myocardial infarction. *Heart* 2000; **83**: 726–30.

Stone GW. Angioplasty strategies in ST-segment elevation myocardial infarction: Part I: primary percutaneous coronary intervention. *Circulation* 2008; **118**: 538–51.

Stone GW. Angioplasty strategies in ST-segment elevation myocardial infarction: Part II: intervention after fibrinolytic therapy, integrated treatment recommendations, and future directions. *Circulation* 2008; **118**: 552–66.

Stone GW, et al. Bivalirudin during primary PCI in acute myocardial infarction. *N Engl J Med* 2008; **358**: 2218–30.

Subherwal S, Bach RG, et al. Baseline risk of major bleeding in non ST-segment elevation myocardial infarction: the CRUSADE (Can Rapid risk stratification of Unstable angina patients Suppress ADverse outcomes with Early implementation of the ACC/AHA guidelines) bleeding score. *Circulation* 2009; **119**: 1873–82.

Tackling myocardial infarction. *Drug Ther Bull* 2000; **38**: 17–22.

The Joint ESC/ACCF/AHA/WHF. Universal definition of myocardial infarction. *Eur Heart J* 2007; **28**: 2525–38.

The Magnesium in Coronaries (MAGIC) Trial Investigators. Early administration of intravenous magnesium to high risk patients with acute myocardial infarction in the Magnesium in Coronaries (MAGIC) trial. *Lancet* 2002; **360**: 1189–96.

The Oasis-6 investigators. Effects of fondaparinux on mortality and reinfarction in patients with acute ST-segment elevation myocardial infarction: the OASIS-6 randomized trial. *JAMA* 2006; **295**(13): 1519–30.

The Task Force on the Management of ST-Segment Elevation Acute Myocardial Infarction of the European Society of Cardiology. Management of acute myocardial infarction in patients presenting with persistent ST-segment elevation. *Eur Heart J* 2008; **29**: 2909–45.

The Task Force for the Diagnosis and Treatment of Non-ST-Segment Elevation Acute Coronary Syndromes of the European Society of Cardiology. Guidelines for the diagnosis and treatment of non-ST-segment elevation acute coronary syndromes. *Eur Heart J* 2007; **28**: 1598–1660.

Topal EJ. Acute myocardial infarction: thrombolysis. *Heart* 2000; **83**: 122–6.

Van der Werf F, Vahanian A, Gulba DC, et al. Selection of reperfusion therapy for individual patients with evolving myocardial infarction. *Eur Heart J* 1997; **18**: 1371–81.

Wallentin L, et al. Ticagrelor versus clopidogrel in patients with acute coronary syndromes. *N Engl J Med* 2009; **361**: 1045–57.

White D. Evolution of the definition of myocardial infarction: what are the implications of a new universal definition? *Heart* 2008; **94**: 679–84.

White D, Chew D. Acute myocardial infarction. *Lancet* 2008; **372**: 570–84.

Wiegers SE, St John Sutton M. When should ACE inhibitors or warfarin be discontinued after myocardial infarction? *Heart* 2000; **84**: 361–2.

Williams SG, Wright DJ, Tan LB. Management of cardiogenic shock complicating acute myocardial infarction: towards evidence based medical practice. *Heart* 2000; **83**: 621–6.

Wiviott SD, et al. Prasugrel versus clopidogrel in patients with acute coronary syndromes. *N Engl J Med* 2007; **357**: 2001–15.

Yusuf S, Mehta SR, Chrolavicius S, et al. Comparison of fondaparinux and enoxaparin in acute coronary syndromes. *N Engl J Med* 2006; **354**:1464–76.

Zijlstra F. Acute myocardial infarction: primary PCI. *Heart* 2001; **85**: 705–9.

CHAPTER 2

RESUSCITATION

BACKGROUND

Epidemiology and physiology

Cardiovascular disease is the leading cause of death in the UK, with more than 300 000 victims each year. Sudden cardiac death represents approximately 25–30 per cent of all cardiovascular death, claiming an estimated 70 000–90 000 lives each year.

Although the causes of cardiac arrest are numerous (Table 2.1), most events in adults occur as a result of ischaemic heart disease. A number of studies have shown a circadian pattern of cardiac arrest with the majority of events occurring in the morning hours (6 a.m. to 12 noon) and a low

Table 2.1 Causes of VF/pulseless VT, asystole and pulseless electrical activity (PEA)

Causes of ventricular fibrillation
Reversible triggers
Acute myocardial infarction/ischaemia
Electrolyte disturbances (hypokalaemia, hyperkalaemia, hypocalcaemia, hypomagnesaemia, metabolic acidosis, etc.)
Drugs (antiarrhythmics, phenothiazines, tricyclic antidepressants, digoxin toxicity, etc.)
Illicit drug use, e.g. cocaine, amphetamines, ecstasy (see Chapter 8)
Commotio cordis (see Chapter 10, cardiac trauma)
Electric shock

Structural heart disease

Coronary artery disease

- Atherosclerotic
- Non-atherosclerotic (Prinzmetal angina, anomalous origin of coronary artery, etc.)

Cardiomyopathies

Valvular heart disease

Myocarditis

Congenital heart disease

Arrhythmogenic right ventricular dysplasia

Primary pulmonary hypertension

Infiltrative heart disease (amyloidosis, sarcoidosis, tumour)

Structurally normal heart

Wolff–Parkinson–White syndrome

Long QT syndromes

Brugada syndrome

Idiopathic VT/VF

Causes of asystole

Heart block

Myocardial infarction

Hypoxia

Drugs (antiarrhythmics, beta-blockers, verapamil) especially with pre-existing sinus node disease

Causes of pulseless electrical activity

'4 Hs and 4 Ts'

Hypoxia

Hypovolaemia

Hypo/hyperkalaemia and other metabolic disorders

Hypothermia

Tension pneumothorax

Tamponade

Toxic/therapeutic disorders

Thromboembolic and mechanical obstruction

incidence at night. Some data also suggest a late afternoon peak between 4 p.m. and 7 p.m. A seasonal variation in cardiac arrest is also recognized with an increased number of cases occurring during the winter months. Resuscitation after cardiopulmonary arrest is effective in only one in five patients with about a third of long-term survivors having apparent motor or cognitive deficits.

By far the most commonly encountered rhythm is ventricular fibrillation (VF) or pulseless ventricular tachycardia (VT) occurring in more than 50 per cent of cases. With time, VF deteriorates from coarse VF to fine VF and eventually to asystole. The prognosis is less favourable for non-VF/VT rhythms. Independent predictors of mortality during follow-up include increased age (>65 years), the presence of heart failure and cardiac arrest not related to an acute coronary syndrome (ACS).

After a cardiac arrest, the only interventions that have been proven to improve long-term survival are basic life support and early defibrillation [immediate commencement of cardiopulmonary resuscitation (CPR) confers a 2.7-fold increase in the rate of survival]. Therefore, the key to a successful outcome is dependent on initiation of a rapid sequence of events with minimal delay (Figure 2.1). Ideally, the goal of in-hospital defibrillation should be a collapse–shock interval of less than 3 minutes. Although data from randomized controlled trials are limited, techniques for CPR have been standardized in recent years, and the guidelines in this chapter are based on those published by the Resuscitation Council (UK) and the European Resuscitation Council (ERC).

The major role of CPR is to provide some blood flow to both the myocardium and central nervous system to allow for successful defibrillation and resuscitation, and to preserve long-term organ function. Although a number of theories have been proposed, the mechanism by

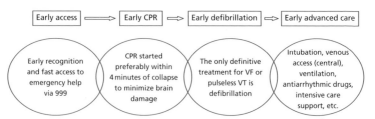

Figure 2.1 The key to a successful resuscitation outcome is dependent on a rapid sequence of events with minimal delay.

which external chest compression provides an artificial circulation is not fully known. Even when performed optimally, chest compression does not achieve more than 30 per cent of the normal cardiac output. One of the most important concepts in understanding the physiology of CPR is that of coronary perfusion pressure. Coronary perfusion pressure is defined as the difference between the aortic diastolic pressure and the right atrial pressure (the venous return of myocardial flow is through the great cardiac vein, coronary sinus and eventually the right atrium; therefore, an increase in right atrial pressure may impede venous run-off from the myocardial capillary bed). The majority of coronary flow occurs during artificial diastole or the chest relaxation phase of CPR, and is dependent on the coronary perfusion pressure. Experimental studies have shown that the larger the coronary perfusion pressure, the greater the coronary blood flow, and the greater the chance for a successful outcome. The coronary perfusion pressure can be optimized by increasing the peripheral vascular tone using vasoconstrictors such as adrenaline, or by increasing the number of chest compressions per minute. A compression rate of 100 per minute is currently recommended by the ERC, partly due to concerns that higher rates may be physically too exhausting for members of the arrest team.

During cardiac arrest and CPR, a severe mixed acidosis can develop. A reduction in alveolar gaseous exchange because of an increase in dead space and a decrease in lung compliance (due to pulmonary oedema) can lead to respiratory acidosis. The combination of circulatory collapse and poor tissue perfusion can result in marked metabolic acidosis. Severe acidosis is negatively inotropic, causes electrolyte disturbances and can cause intractable arrhythmias and a poor resuscitation outcome.

THE ABC OF RESUSCITATION AND SPECIFIC INTERVENTIONS

The ABC of resuscitation begins with basic life support and the establishment of an adequate airway (A), breathing (B) and circulation (C). The purpose of basic life support is to maintain adequate ventilation and circulation until advanced techniques can be applied to reverse the underlying cause of the arrest. It is assumed that a sound knowledge in basic life support already exists, and therefore this chapter concentrates mainly on management issues and interventions during advanced life support.

Airway
A quick inspection of the oropharynx should be performed, and any obstructions such as food or loose dentures should be removed. Tight-fitting dentures should be left as it helps support the soft palate. Manoeuvres

such as the head tilt, chin lift and jaw thrust can be used to ensure that the tongue and soft tissues do not obstruct the airway. A variety of airway adjuncts are now available on most resuscitation trolleys and include facial masks, Guedel airways (an estimate of the size may be obtained by selecting an airway with a length corresponding to the vertical distance between the incisor tooth and the angle of the jaw) and nasopharyngeal tubes (the diameter size in adults is usually 6–7 mm or the diameter of the little finger). The tip of a nasopharyngeal tube should be visible in the pharynx behind the tongue. For more skilled and experienced staff, the insertion of a laryngeal mask or, ideally, an endotracheal tube can be attempted.

Breathing

It is important to look, listen and feel for breath sounds and chest movements. In any patient in whom breathing is inadequate or absent, artificial ventilation must be commenced as soon as possible. Oxygenation of the patient is the primary objective and the highest concentration of oxygen available should be administered. This can be achieved by using a mask with a reservoir bag, which can deliver inspired oxygen concentrations of 85 per cent at flow rates of 10–15 L/min. Tidal volumes of 400–600 mL are adequate to make the chest rise and are less likely to cause gastric insufflation and aspiration. Between 1.5 and 2 seconds should be spent in the inspiratory phase.

Circulation

Until now, previous resuscitation guidelines have required the absence of a carotid pulse to diagnose cardiac arrest and start CPR. However, times in excess of 30 seconds are required to achieve an accuracy of 95 per cent. As a consequence, current guidelines have de-emphasized the carotid pulse as the sole criterion for starting CPR, and include the search for signs of a circulation such as chest wall movement and breathing. If there is no circulation, then chest compressions should be commenced. The heel of one hand should be placed in the middle of the lower half of the sternum, the fingers should be off the chest and the other hand is brought down to rest on the back of the hand with the fingers interlocked. Vertical downward pressure is applied to depress the sternum 4–5 cm and then the pressure is released. A compression rate of 100 per minute using a compression to ventilation ratio of 30:2 is now recommended for single and multiple rescuers when ventilating non-invasively (bag and mask). Once intubated, ventilation should continue at approximately 12 breaths/min with chest compression maintained uninterrupted for ventilation. Uninterrupted chest compression results in substantially higher mean coronary perfusion pressure.

Defibrillation

The only definitive treatment for VF or pulseless VT is defibrillation. Although these rhythms are initially readily treatable, the chances of successful defibrillation diminish rapidly with time and decline by 7–10 per cent per minute. In the case of a witnessed arrest especially when a shockable rhythm has been identified, it is reasonable to attempt a precordial thump. The thump delivers a small amount of kinetic energy, which may be adequate to convert a fibrillating myocardium. All reported cases of successful precordial thump occurred within 10 seconds of VF/VT. If precordial thump is not successful or if VF/VT is more prolonged then electrical cardioversion is required. Often, patients are not monitored and the duration of VF/VT is unknown, in this case chest compressions should be initiated first until the rhythm is determined. Experimental studies have shown that interruption in chest compressions is associated with a lower chance of survival. In addition, interruptions in chest compression reduce the chance of successfully converting VF to another rhythm. Therefore, unless the patient is monitored and defibrillation can be achieved immediately after collapse, chest compressions should be started and maintained until defibrillation is possible. Following defibrillation chest compressions should be continued as delay in checking for a pulse may further compromise the myocardium if a perfusing rhythm has not been restored.

Shocks are initially started at between 150 J and 360 J with a biphasic device. Biphasic shocks involve the polarity of the current being reversed part way through the delivery of a shock, as a result the defibrillation threshold is lowered and the shock energy required for successful defibrillation is reduced. Monophasic defibrillators are being phased out as they are less efficient at terminating VF/VT. If they are used they should be set to 360 J from the outset. The paddles should be applied firmly to the chest wall with water-based gel pads between them and the skin. The pressure applied should be approximately 8 kg of force and the correct positions are shown in Figure 2.2a. The use of hands-free self-adhesive pads allows for safer operation by allowing the operator to discharge the device without leaning over the patient. They also allow for quick identification of rhythm and therefore quicker defibrillation than using standard electrodes. If defibrillation is unsuccessful in the anterolateral position, then further attempts in the anteroposterior position (Figure 2.2b) and/or a different

Anterior-lateral electrode position for defibrillation and/or transcutaneous cardiac pacing

Anterior-posterior electrode position for defibrillation and/or transcutaneous cardiac pacing

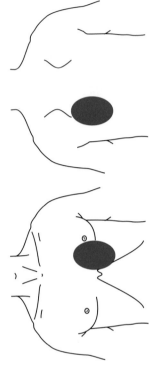

One electrode is placed to the left of the lower sternal border (corresponding to V2 and V3 ECG electrode). The other electrode is placed beneath the scapula, lateral to the spine on the left, at the same level as the anterior electrode.

(b)

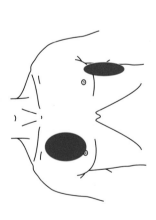

One electrode is placed to the right of the upper sternum below the clavicle.
The other electrode is placed at the level of the fifth intercostal space in the anterior axillary line (corresponding to V5–V6 ECG electrode).

(a)

Figure 2.2 Paddle positions for anterior-lateral and anterior-posterior defibrillation.

defibrillator are worth trying. The positions of the positive and negative paddles do not matter when defibrillating.

In patients with permanent pacemakers, defibrillation in the anteroposterior position is preferable, even though modern pacemakers are fitted with protection circuits. When defibrillation is attempted, ensure that the electrodes are placed at least 12–15 cm from the pacemaker unit.

Pacing

Pacing can often be life saving, especially in situations where bradycardia preceded the cardiac arrest or where bradycardia is associated with haemodynamic intolerance following successful resuscitation. Pacing can be attempted non-invasively or invasively, depending on the equipment available and/or the experience of the operator.

Non-invasive (transcutaneous) pacing

Transcutaneous pacing can be easily applied, requires minimum training and avoids the risks of central venous cannulation. Many defibrillators are now equipped with external pacing facilities and it is important for those involved in managing cardiac arrest to familiarize themselves with this option. Pacing is usually carried out through self-adhesive gel pads which can also be used for defibrillation if necessary. When used for pacing, the device often additionally requires a 3-lead ECG (electrocardiogram) to be attached. The ECG gain is adjusted to ensure sensing of any intrinsic QRS complexes. The demand mode is selected and the pacing rate set to 60–90 bpm. The pacing current is set at the lowest setting and the pacemaker turned on. The current is then slowly increased, observing the patient, and monitored until electrical capture is seen. As the current increases, the skeletal muscles contract and a pacing spike is seen on the monitor. Electrical capture is recognized by wide QRS complex and a broad T wave. A current range of 50–100 mA is usually sufficient (Figure 2.3). The presence of a palpable pulse ensures electrical capture results in mechanical capture (myocardial contraction). Failure to achieve mechanical capture in the presence of good electrical capture indicates non-functional myocardium. Patients often require sedation with an IV benzodiazepine (Diazemuls) as the procedure can be painful. Transcutaneous pacing is only a temporary measure until transvenous pacing can be instituted.

Transvenous pacing (box 2.1)

The resuscitation trolley should always be present and venous access available. Bradycardia, asystole and ventricular tachyarrhythmias are

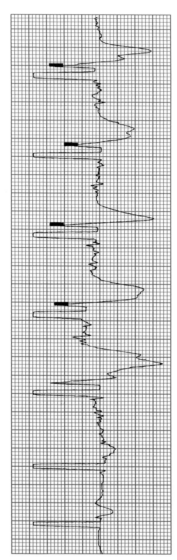

Figure 2.3 Non-invasive transcutaneous pacing. The first two pacing spikes are not followed by a QRST wave complex and therefore signify failure to capture. The remaining pacing spikes demonstrate ventricular capture. It is important to ensure that electrical capture is associated with mechanical capture by the presence of a palpable pulse.

often induced during the procedure, and therefore atropine, isoprenaline and lidocaine should be readily at hand. The commonest route for placing a temporary wire is usually the right subclavian vein (the left side is then available for a permanent implant if required). The risk of vascular access site complications can be reduced by using the femoral vein, with the additional advantages that haemostasis can easily be secured by pressure if bleeding occurs, and the requirement for wire manipulation during placement is usually minimal.

Box 2.1 Indications for temporary transvenous cardiac pacing

Emergency/acute

Acute myocardial infarction
- Asystole
- Symptomatic bradycardia (sinus bradycardia with hypotension and Mobitz type 1 second degree AV block with hypotension not responsive to atropine)
- Bilateral bundle branch block (alternating BBB or RBBB with alternating LAHB/LPHB)
- New or indeterminate age bifascicular block with first degree AV block (trifascicular block)
- Mobitz type 2 second degree AV block
- Overdrive suppression of tachyarrhythmias

Bradycardia not associated with acute myocardial infarction
- Asystole
- Second or third degree AV block with haemodynamic compromise or syncope at rest
- Ventricular tachyarrhythmias secondary to bradycardia

Elective
- Support for procedures that may promote bradycardia
- General anaesthesia with:
  - second or third degree AV block
  - intermittent AV block
  - first degree AV block with bifascicular block
  - first degree AV block and LBBB
- Cardiac surgery
  - aortic surgery
  - tricuspid surgery
  - ventricular septal defect closure
  - ostium primum repair

BBB, bundle branch block; LAHB, left anterior hemiblock; LPHB, left posterior hemiblock; RBBB, right bundle branch block.

A sheath with a non-return valve should be placed in the vein using a Seldinger technique, to allow easy manipulation of the wire. A size 5F bipolar pacing wire is appropriate in most cases. A working pacing box (pulse generator) must be ready before inserting the wire. When using the subclavian approach (with a standard 20–30° curve on the wire tip), the wire is advanced into the right atrium under fluoroscopic control and rotated until it points downwards and to the patient's left. Advancing across the tricuspid valve will often induce ventricular ectopics, which usually settle rapidly and require no treatment. If difficulty is encountered in crossing the tricuspid valve, changing the curve at the wire tip usually helps. If this fails, fashioning the electrode into a loop in the right atrium by pointing the lead tip to the right cardiac border may be successful. The electrode is twisted clockwise or anticlockwise until the tip lies near the tricuspid valve. Slight withdrawal of the electrode at this stage will allow the tip to flick through the valve into the right ventricle. The electrode should never be advanced if resistance is encountered: rather, the electrode should be withdrawn slightly, rotated and then carefully advanced again. When using the femoral approach, the curve on the wire tip should be directed towards the midline as the wire enters the right atrium. As the wire is subsequently advanced it usually easily crosses the tricuspid valve.

The best position for the pacing wire is usually with the tip in the right ventricular apex, to the left of the midline and with the tip of the wire pointing inferiorly on screening (if the wire is directed to the left, towards the left shoulder, it may be in the coronary sinus and often will not capture at an acceptable threshold). There should be enough slack in the loop of the electrode to allow for changes in posture and deep inspiration, but not so much as to allow the tip to displace either in the right atrium or the pulmonary artery. The wire is then attached to the connecting leads and pacing box.

To test the threshold, the pacing box is first set to the demand mode, then the pacing rate set at 5–10 bpm faster than the patient's intrinsic rate. The output is set at 3 V; this should result in a paced rhythm. The amplitude of the voltage is slowly turned down until capture is lost. Acceptable stimulation thresholds are below 1 V, although higher levels may be acceptable if the patient is elderly, has had an inferior infarct, or if several sites have been tried, all with relatively high thresholds. The stability of the pacing wire is checked during deep breathing, coughing and sniffing. If capture is lost then a more stable position should be sought. Once the threshold has been ascertained, the output voltage should be set at three times the threshold or 3 V, whichever is higher. This compensates for subsequent threshold elevations due to inflammation and oedema at the electrode–tissue interface. If in sinus rhythm, a back-up rate of 50/min is set. If there is heart block or bradycardia, the rate is normally set at 70–80/min.

The wire is sutured firmly with a loop formed externally to minimize the chance of inadvertent lead displacement. Finally, a chest x-ray is obtained to exclude any complications.

Temporary venous pacemakers should be checked at least once daily for pacing threshold, evidence of infections around venous access sites, integrity of connections, and battery status of the external generator. Underlying rhythm should also be assessed and recorded at these checks. Pacing thresholds are checked by increasing the pacing rate to obtain continuous pacing, then progressively decreasing the output voltage until capture is lost. A sudden increase in the threshold usually indicates the need for repositioning.

ARRHYTHMIA ALGORITHMS

Shockable rhythms (VF/pulseless VT)

This is recognized on the cardiac monitor by the presence of chaotic fibrillation waves, due to wandering cardiac electrical activity along continuously changing pathways (Figure 2.4a, Box 2.1) or a broad complex tachycardia (Figure 2.4b). Defibrillation with a biphasic shock is the definitive treatment for VF (Figure 2.5). The likelihood of survival decreases 10 per cent for each minute of time after the onset of uncorrected VF. Defibrillation should be performed as soon as the diagnosis of VF is considered, with an initial shock of 150 J to 360 J, followed by chest compressions. If pulseless electrical activity develops, the non-shockable algorithm is followed. If VF persists, CPR is maintained for 2 minutes, followed by assessment of rhythm and further shocks if indicated (Figure 2.5). During CPR, an adequate airway and oxygenation (intubating the patient only if trained or experienced) are ensured, intravenous access obtained, and adrenaline 1 mg administered every 3–5 minutes. Adrenaline works principally as a vasoconstrictor (α-agonist effect) to increase the efficiency of basic life support, not as an adjuvant to defibrillation. Adrenaline 2–3 mg (made up to a volume of 10 mL using sterile water) can be given via the tracheal tube. This should

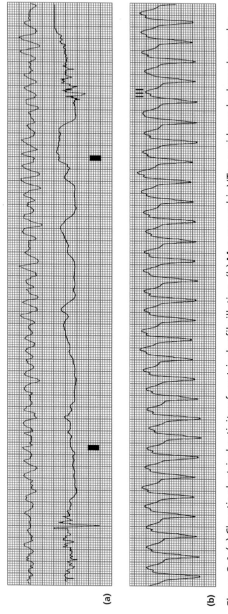

Figure 2.4 (a) Chaotic electrical activity of ventricular fibrillation. (b) Monomorphic VT: a rapid regular broad complex tachycardia.

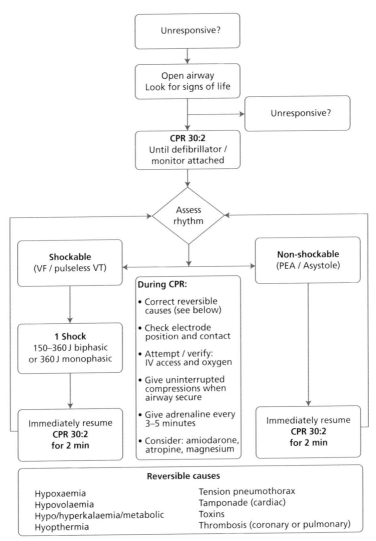

Figure 2.5 Cardiac arrest algorithm based on the European Resuscitation Council and the Resuscitation Council (UK).

then be followed by at least five ventilations to disperse the drug into the peripheral bronchial tree and aid absorption.

Recent studies suggest that amiodarone may be superior to lidocaine in cardioverting shock-resistant VF. In addtion there is evidence that amiodarone increases the chance of survival to hospital for shock-resistant VF. Therefore, it is now recommended that amiodarone be used as the first-choice antifibrillatory agent. A dose of 300 mg IV should be administered if VF/VT persists after three shocks. Lidocaine can be used if amiodarone is not available though it should not be given if amiodarone has already been used due to potential pro-arrhythmic effects of multiple drugs. Drug doses and infusion regimens are discussed in Appendix A.

Non-shockable rhythms

These rhythms usually have a poor outcome unless a reversible cause can be found and rapidly treated. The right side of the resuscitation algorithm (Figure 2.5) should be followed.

Asystole

This is recognized by the total absence of any ventricular electrical activity on the cardiac monitor. Causes are summarized in Box 2.1. The gain setting on the monitor is set to 1 mV and the leads and electrical connections are secured. Where possible, an additional lead should be viewed so as to avoid missing a potentially reversible arrhythmia (fine ventricular fibrillation). If in doubt, treatment is with defibrillation as in VF/pulseless VT. Basic life support should be commenced for 2 minutes, during which time advanced airway and ventilation techniques are performed, intravenous access gained and adrenaline 1 mg given. Atropine 3 mg IV or 6 mg via the tracheal tube (made up to a volume of at least 10 mL of sterile water) is administered. The monitor should be closely inspected for the presence of atrial activity (P waves), which may suggest complete heart block with ventricular asystole. This may respond to external (transcutaneous) or transvenous pacing depending on the skills and equipment available. If asystole persists, CPR is continued with the administration of adrenaline 1 mg every 3–5 minutes. The administration of higher-dose adrenaline as a single bolus is no longer recommended.

Pulseless electrical activity

This is recognized by the presence of an ECG rhythm compatible with a cardiac output in the setting of a cardiac arrest. The commonest cause of sudden, unexpected development of pulseless electrical activity (PEA) following an acute STEMI is rupture of the ventricular free wall. Successful resuscitation in this situation is very rare. Other important causes to consider are summarized in Box 2.1. The best chance of survival is the early diagnosis and treatment of the conditions detailed in Box 2.1. Having instituted basic and advanced life support, and administered any specific therapy for the above conditions, IV adrenaline 1 mg is given every 3–5 minutes.

EARLY POST-RESUSCITATION CARE

Immediately after an arrest, blood gases, electrolytes, cardiac-specific enzymes, full blood count and ECG are checked, and any problems treated. For instance:

- Hypoxia is usually present, so high concentrations of oxygen should be given. Oxygen saturation is monitored with pulse oximetry, ensuring a saturation of >93 per cent.

- Serum potassium is maintained above 4 mmol/L and magnesium above 2 mmol/L. If potassium is above 6 mmol/L, 10 mL of 10 per cent calcium chloride is given IV over 5 minutes, followed by 50 mL of 50 per cent dextrose and 10 units of Actrapid (insulin) to stabilize the myocardium and correct hyperkalaemia.

- If the pH is less than 7.1 or the base excess ≤10 mmol/L, giving bicarbonate (8.4 per cent) in 25-mL boluses should be considered to maintain a pH of 7.3–7.5.

- Consider the need for antiarrhythmic drug therapy to limit the risk of further arrhythmia.

- Hyperglycaemia should be controlled with an insulin sliding-scale regimen.

- Hypoglycaemia should be treated with a bolus of 20 mL of 50 per cent dextrose or glucose solution IV.

- Persistent cardiac ischaemia that may have precipitated the cardiac arrest should be looked for and treated. In particular VT/VF that is ischaemia driven may respond to the use of an intra-aortic balloon pump.

- A portable chest x-ray should be arranged and any pneumothorax treated.

- Left ventricular failure and hypotension should be treated, if present. If hypotension persists consider a pulmonary artery catheter to guide optimal fluid and inotropic therapy.

- The patient should be catheterized and urine output monitored.

- The nervous system should be examined and neurological function documented using the Glasgow Coma Scale.

- The patient should be examined to ensure that there is no other medical or surgical intervention requiring immediate management.

- A comprehensive history should be obtained, including a family history from available witnesses. The possibility of overdoses and other non-primary cardiac disease (such as hypothermia, cerebrovascular accidents, subarachnoid haemorrhages, etc., see Box 2.1) should be excluded.

There are no definitive data as to when to discontinue intravenous antiarrhythmic drug infusions. It is common clinical practice to continue the infusion for a minimal of 24–48 hours and to discontinue the infusion provided there is no arrhythmic recurrence. For patients with refractory ventricular arrhythmias, high-dose beta-blockade coupled with atrial or dual chamber pacemaker therapy, and light anaesthesia together with muscle relaxation and artificial ventilation, may be life saving. Urgent referral for coronary revascularization or electrophysiological testing should be considered.

Following a successful resuscitation, most patients will regain consciousness rapidly. Hypoxia must be avoided after resuscitation, and assisted ventilation should be used if there is a reasonable chance of recovery. The patient who remains unconscious and dependent on assisted ventilation should be transferred to the intensive care unit after close liaison with the anaesthetist. The decision to withdraw ventilatory support should be made by the most senior member of the medical/anaesthetic team. The opinions of other members of the medical and nursing team, the patient (if previously known) and their relatives should be taken into consideration before making a final decision.

If asystole or PEA persists after 25 minutes of resuscitation in a normothermic adult without drug toxicity, then success is unlikely and the attempt should probably be abandoned. If VF persists at this point, the situation is still potentially reversible, and it may be worth persisting with attempts at resuscitation. Pupillary dilatation should not be used as a reason for discontinuing resuscitation, as this can be drug induced. When hypothermia is present, attempts to revive the patient should be continued for longer, probably until core temperature is above 36°C and arterial pH and potassium are normal. It is well documented that full recovery can occur with resuscitation attempts of up to 9 hours.

LATE POST-RESUSCITATION CARE

Following a cardiac arrest, patients should be thoroughly investigated and appropriate therapy directed to minimize the risk of recurrence (Box 2.1). Reversible triggers such as ACS, electrolyte disturbances, drugs (both prescribed and illicit) should be excluded. These can usually be diagnosed from the history, biochemical tests (including toxicology screens and cardiac enzymes) and serial ECGs. Structural heart disease can be excluded with echocardiograms, left and right heart cardiac catheterization (including right ventriculogram and myocardial biopsy) and magnetic resonance imaging (MRI). Patients with structurally normal hearts should be investigated with a 24–48-hour Holter monitor, exercise stress testing and possible programmed electrophysiological stimulation. Particular attention should be paid to the response of the QT interval during Holter monitoring and stress testing. If no triggering events can be identified, then patients should be considered for an implantable cardioverter defibrillator.

Where there is a family history of sudden cardiac death, the patient's family should be screened with an ECG, Holter monitor, echocardiogram and stress testing. Genetic screening for some of the inherited syndromes can also be carried out in some centres.

NEW DEVELOPMENTS

Alternative techniques to standard manual CPR have been developed to improve perfusion during CPR. Active compression–decompression CPR (ACD-CPR) is performed with a portable device equipped with suction cup to actively lift the anterior chest during decompression. This decreases intrathoracic pressure, enhancing venous return for the next compression. Randomized studies have shown equivocal benefit using this technique, and therefore it is not recommended for routine use at present. However, these devices may be advantageous in situations where delivering adequate chest compressions is difficult, such as during transport. They have also been used in several cases that allowed patients to undergo CT scanning or even coronary angiography without interrupting CPR.

The major determinant of survival in patients with VF and pulseless VT is the time taken for defibrillation. Consequently, there has been a natural progression to make defibrillators more available. The development and easy applicability of automatic external defibrillators have strengthened this view. Once a cardiac arrest has been diagnosed, the electrodes of the system are attached to the chest using the standard positions. The device is able to recognize VF and deliver defibrillatory shocks if required. Instructions are provided automatically on the screen and some models reinforce these instructions with synthesized voice messages. An override facility is available if one wants to use it as a manual defibrillator. These devices can be used by the public and require minimal training. Consequently, in some countries, these devices are now deployed in public locations such as airports, commercial aircraft, train stations and casinos. Recently, the US Food and Drug Administration has approved a vest-like defibrillator device that can be worn under clothing, rather than being implanted in the chest. The vest contains an electrode belt that is applied to the chest and monitors the heart rhythm. If an abnormal life-threatening heart rhythm is detected, and the patient loses consciousness, the device administers an electrical shock.

KEY POINTS

- CPR is a dynamic subject and therefore all health care staff involved in patient care should be trained and kept up to date with advanced life support protocols.

- The most commonly encountered rhythm during a cardiac arrest is VF or pulseless VT.

- The prognosis is less favourable for non-shockable rhythms unless a reversible cause is present.

- The only interventions that have been shown to improve long-term survival are basic life support and early defibrillation.

- Careful post-resuscitation care is essential to maximize the chances of a full recovery.

KEY REFERENCES

Adgey AAJ, Johnston PW. Approaches to modern management of cardiac arrest. *Heart* 1998; **80**: 397–401.

Berg RA, Sanders AB, Kern KB, et al. Adverse hemodynamic effects of interrupting chest compressions for rescue breathing during cardiopulmonary resuscitation for ventricular fibrillation cardiac arrest. *Circulation* 2001; **104**: 2465–70.

Dorian P, Cass D, Schwartz B, Cooper R, Gelaznikas R, Barr A. Amiodarone as compared with lidocaine for shock-resistant ventricular fibrillation. *N Engl J Med* 2002; **346**: 884–90.

Eftestol T, Sunde K, Steen PA. Effects of interrupting precordial compressions on the calculated probability of defibrillation success during out-of-hospital cardiac arrest. *Circulation* 2002; **105**: 2270–3.

Eisenberg MS, Mengert TJ. Cardiac resuscitation. *N Engl J Med* 2001; 344: 1304–13.

Gammage MD. Temporary cardiac pacing. *Heart* 2000; **83**: 715–20.

Gilbert M, Busund R, Skagseth A, Nilsen P, Solbo JP. Resuscitation from accidental hypothermia of 13.7°C with circulatory arrest. *Lancet* 2000; **355**: 375–6.

Handley AJ. Teaching hand placement for chest compression – a simpler technique. *Resuscitation* 2002; **53**: 29–36.

Kern KB. Cardiopulmonary resuscitation physiology. *ACC Curr J Rev* 1997; **6**: 11–13.

Kudenchuk PJ, Cobb LA, Copass MK, et al. Amiodarone for resuscitation after out of hospital cardiac arrest due to ventricular fibrillation. *N Engl J Med* 1999; **341**: 871–8.

Nademanee K, Taylor R, Bailey WE, Rieders DE, Kosar EM. Treating electrical storm sympathetic blockade versus advanced cardiac life support-guided therapy. *Circulation* 2000; **102**: 742–7.

Peckova M, Fahrenbruch CE, Cobb LA, Hallstrom AP. Circadian variations in the occurrence of cardiac arrest. Initial and repeat episodes. *Circulation* 1998; **98**: 31–9.

Resuscitation Council (UK). *Advanced Life Support Course Provider Manual.* London: Resuscitation Council, 2005.

Wik L, Hansen TB, Fylling F, et al. Delaying defibrillation to give basic cardiopulmonary resuscitation to patients with out-of-hospital ventricular fibrillation: a randomized trial. *JAMA* 2003; **289**: 1389–95.

ARRHYTHMIAS

BACKGROUND

The management of cardiac arrhythmias complicating acute coronary syndrome (ACS) is dealt with in Chapter 1. This chapter deals with the management of arrhythmias that occur as a complication of other cardiac and medical disorders. Optimal treatment of these arrhythmias depends on two principles:

- inspecting the electrocardiogram (ECG) and reviewing the clinical presentation to establish the diagnosis. This provides information about arrhythmia mechanism and guides treatment selection.

- assessing the effect of the arrhythmia. Patients with good cardiac function will often tolerate arrhythmias without major haemodynamic compromise. Patients with coexistent cardiac impairment may be severely compromised by an arrhythmia. Tachyarrhythmias associated with major haemodynamic compromise usually require urgent cardioversion. Bradyarrhythmias associated with major haemodynamic compromise often require pacing. Patients with better tolerated arrhythmias can be treated with drug therapy.

If there is any doubt about diagnosis or treatment, **a senior colleague should be consulted for advice.**

The symptoms produced by the onset of an arrhythmia are highly variable. In an individual with no cardiac disease, an arrhythmia may be asymptomatic. A rapid tachyarrhythmia often produces palpitations. In patients with cardiac disease, arrhythmia-related reduction in cardiac output and coronary perfusion may lead to ischaemic chest pain, heart failure and disturbed consciousness.

It is useful to classify tachycardias according to whether the ECG QRS complexes are narrow or broad.

Narrow-complex tachyarrhythmias usually arise from above the level of the bundle of His. In most cases, ventricular activation occurs via the normal conduction system, hence the narrow QRS configuration. This group can itself be subdivided into two groups, depending on whether they arise from the atrial myocardium (atrial fibrillation [AF], atrial flutter and atrial tachycardia) or a mechanism involving the atrioventricular (AV) node (atrioventricular nodal re-entry tachycardia [AVNRT] and atrioventricular re-entry tachycardia [AVRT] accessory pathways). The commonest narrow-complex tachyarrhythmias are AF, atrial flutter and AVNRT.

Broad-complex tachyarrhythmias usually arise from the ventricles, although some ventricular tachyarrhythmias arise high in the bundle of His and can be relatively narrow. In a minority of cases, tachyarrhythmias arising from above the bundle of His can be associated with a broad QRS complex: abnormal slow ventricular activation occurs in those with pre-existing or rate-related bundle branch block, and in some patients with an accessory pathway. Because of this overlap, QRS duration is not a totally reliable guide to the site of origin of an arrhythmia, and additional information obtained from careful inspection of all features of the ECG, previous ECGs and ECGs in sinus rhythm is required before a diagnosis can be reached.

Antiarrhythmic drug therapy has important limitations. The available agents are of limited efficacy, and a drug prescribed in the correct dose for an appropriate indication may fail to work. The available drugs may themselves be pro-arrhythmic, and may also have many unwanted side effects, including causing impairment of myocardial contractility, gastrointestinal and central nervous system disturbances. The available drugs can be categorized using the Vaughan–Williams classification, which provides information on the drugs' electrophysiological effects:

- **CLASS I:** these agents have membrane-stabilizing properties, slowing sodium transport during myocyte depolarization, and can act on the atria, ventricles or conduction tissue.
- **CLASS II:** these agents block cardiac beta-receptors and act predominantly on the sinus and AV nodes (although there is

also some membrane-stabilizing effect in the atria and ventricles).

- **CLASS III:** these agents act on myocyte potassium channels, prolong the duration of the action potential and can act on the atria, ventricles or conduction system.
- **CLASS IV:** these agents block calcium channels, and act predominantly on the sinus and AV nodes.

Some drugs have more than one class of action, and others such as adenosine and digoxin cannot be classified using this simple system. Because of the complex nature of these drugs and the potential to induce a wide range of adverse effects, it is important to become familiar with the use of a small number of front-line drugs. Polypharmacy should be avoided; if the first-line therapy fails, a senior colleague should be contacted for advice before using a second drug. The onset of an arrhythmia is often associated with problems such as heart failure, pulmonary infection or embolism, thyroid disturbance, hypoxia, electrolyte imbalance or drug administration. It is important to look for and treat correctable factors that may initiate or perpetuate an arrhythmia.

ATRIAL FIBRILLATION

Background

AF is the most common cardiac arrhythmia (Figure 3.1). The incidence and prevalence of AF increases with age: the prevalence is approximately 9 per cent in patients in their ninth decade.

The development of AF is associated with atrial electrical instability or atrial distension induced by:

- hypertension
- congestive heart failure
- valvular heart disease
- ischaemic heart disease
- pulmonary infection or embolism.

Other less common causes of AF are cardiac trauma (including iatrogenic trauma associated with cardiac surgery), metabolic abnormalities, exposure to toxins (such as alcohol), pericardial disease or systemic infection. In some patients, AF can arise in an otherwise entirely normal heart. This lone AF may be due to small localized areas of electrical instability in the atrium

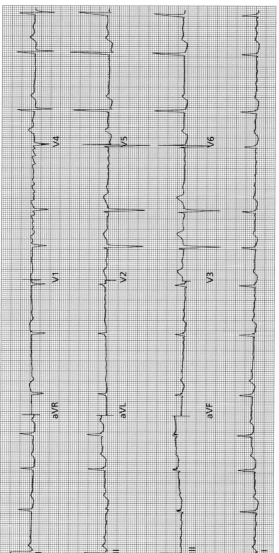

Figure 3.1 Atrial fibrillation is characterized by the absence of P waves and an irregular ventricular rhythm. The 'reverse tick' deformity of the ST segment, associated with digoxin, is best seen here in leads V5 and V6.

(usually close to the pulmonary vein orifices), or increased susceptibility to fluctuations in autonomic neural stimuli to the heart.

Diagnosis and assessment

Regardless of the underlying aetiology, patients with AF develop multiple random wavelets of depolarization in the atrial myocardium. This rapid erratic electrical activity is intermittently conducted to the ventricles via the AV node, producing a rapid, irregularly irregular ventricular rhythm. The onset of AF is often associated with symptoms due to a reduction in cardiac output or the rapid irregular ventricular rhythm causing a sensation of palpitation. The mean resting rate in patients with new onset AF is usually between 110 and 130 bpm. A rate in excess of 150 bpm should raise the suspicion of a hyperadrenergic state (thyrotoxicosis, or fever) or acute blood loss. A very rapid (rate 250 bpm) broad-complex AF is suggestive of the presence of a rapidly anterogradely conducting accessory pathway (Wolff–Parkinson–White syndrome [WPW]).

When AF persists for more than 48 hours, stasis of blood in the fibrillating atrium may lead to clot formation and systemic embolization. The risk of thromboembolism is low in patients with recent-onset (up to 48 hours' duration) AF. In some patients (particularly if cardiac function is normal), the AF will be well tolerated and asymptomatic. The 12-lead ECG of patients with AF will show an absence of P waves, rapid erratic fibrillation activity visible in the baseline between ventricular complexes, and an irregularly irregular ventricular rhythm which usually has a narrow complex QRS configuration. Initially, episodes of AF may be short lived and self-terminating (paroxysmal AF). Repeated episodes, however, lead to adverse changes in atrial electrophysiological and mechanical function, which decrease electrical stability and eventually lead to the development of sustained AF. Episodes of AF that persist for several days rarely terminate spontaneously.

In patient assessment, careful history taking and clinical examination are important. If there is time, a chest x-ray and echocardiogram will also help. Particular importance should be paid to:

- the duration of AF
- the presence of coexistent cardiac disease (such as hypertension, ischaemic heart disease, valvular heart disease or left ventricular dysfunction)
- the effects of AF on patient symptoms, ventricular rate, blood pressure (BP) and cardiac function.

These important features help to guide the selection of appropriate therapy.

Treatment of recent-onset poorly tolerated AF

The onset of AF may be poorly tolerated, producing major symptoms and haemodynamic compromise. Patients with coexistent structural abnormalities (such as valvular heart disease, left ventricular hypertrophy, coronary artery disease or left ventricular dysfunction) or an accessory pathway capable of rapid anterograde conduction are intolerant of AF. When AF is poorly tolerated, many antiarrhythmic drugs are contraindicated or have an unpredictable response. If AF is associated with

- angina or heart failure, or
- rate > 200 bpm, or
- systolic BP < 90 mmHg,
- an accessory pathway

urgent restoration of sinus rhythm by direct current cardioversion (DCC) is the treatment of choice irrespective of the duration of AF. Emergency treatment in this context should not be delayed by the administration of anticoagulants. As long as the AF is of <48 hours' duration, the risk of procedure-related thromboembolism is low. Ideally, if there are no contraindications, heparin should be commenced upon presentation if patients have not been previous anticoagulated to a therapeutic level. Oral anticoagulation should be started if sinus rhythm is not re-established, or for those felt to be at risk of recurrent episodes of AF, or for those at high risk of stroke.

Among patients with permanent AF in whom haemodynamic compromise has recently occurred due to an uncontrolled ventricular response, treatment should focus on rate control.

Treatment of recent-onset well-tolerated AF

In patients with recent-onset (< 48 hours) AF who do not have major symptoms or haemodynamic instability, ideally, electrical cardioversion should be performed. If there is likely to be a delay in performing DCC, AF can be treated with antiarrhythmic drugs. Drugs that act predominantly on the AV node (such as digoxin, beta-blockers and calcium antagonists) are not effective at restoring sinus rhythm. In particular, these agents should **not** be used for patients with WPW syndrome, as they may enhance anterograde conduction via the accessory pathway, potentially resulting in very rapid ventricular rates, hypotension and ventricular fibrillation. Class I or class III drugs that act on the atrial myocardium can restore sinus rhythm in most patients if the drugs are administered early in adequate doses, with the highest success rates achieved by class Ic drugs. If the patient has a structurally normal heart (no significant valve disease, ischaemic heart disease or left ventricular dysfunction) intravenous (IV) flecainide 2 mg/kg (to a maximum of 150 mg) restores sinus rhythm in 90 per cent of patients within 1 hour. The use of flecainide should be avoided if there is any pre-existing structural heart disease, as this will increase the risk of major adverse effects. In a patient with associated structural heart disease, an IV loading dose of amiodarone 300 mg followed by an infusion of 900 mg over 24 hours is safe (see Appendix A), produces rapid slowing of the ventricular rate (due to its beta-blocking effects) and is moderately effective for cardioversion. If pharmacological cardioversion fails, DCC should be performed. Thromboembolism is just as likely to occur following pharmacological, as opposed to electrical, cardioversion. As above, heparin should be commenced immediately the diagnosis is made, followed by warfarin as appropriate.

Treatment of well-tolerated AF of long or unknown duration

If the AF has been present for more than 48 hours (or for an unknown duration), there is a significant thromboembolic risk associated with cardioversion. In these patients, one option is to consider using a strategy of anticoagulation and ventricular rate control, particularly for older patients, those with intolerance to antiarrhythmic agents, and those deemed unsuitable for cardioversion. Anticoagulation may be instituted with heparin followed by warfarin but often warfarin alone is used in the outpatient setting. Digoxin takes several hours to slow the ventricular rate (acting indirectly on the AV node via the autonomic nervous system) and its efficacy is reduced in a hyperadrenergic patient. Intravenous beta-blockers produce rapid rate control regardless of the level of sympathetic tone (e.g. metoprolol or atenolol 5–10 mg according to need and tolerability by slow IV injection is effective in most patients). Intravenous therapy should be followed by adequate oral doses. Where beta-blockers are contraindicated, rate-limiting calcium blockers such as diltiazem or verapamil can be used. If there is coexistent ventricular dysfunction, digoxin (0.125–0.5 mg) is often favoured but gradual introduction of beta-blockers should also be considered for long-term rate control.

Among younger patients, first-time presenters, or those with unacceptable symptoms or with coexistent heart failure, a strategy of rhythm control may be preferred initially. Usually, after a month's anticoagulation, electrical cardioversion can be considered. In certain cases, e.g. where anticoagulation may be associated with a high risk of bleeding, and where facilities and expertise allow, cardioversion can be performed earlier, guided by transoesophageal echocardiography (to exclude the presence of intracardiac thrombus).

Contemporary practice has been influenced following publication of studies (AFFIRM, RACE, and others) that have shown no superiority of rhythm over rate control among older subjects with persistent AF. Indeed, rhythm control was associated with higher rates of embolic stroke, likely related to discontinuation of anticoagulation after regaining sinus rhythm.

Treatment of post-operative AF

Post-operative AF is common, particularly among those undergoing cardiac surgery: it is estimated to occur in up to one-third of patients undergoing coronary artery bypass graft surgery, and is more frequent when valve surgery is undertaken. Older patients, and those with previous episodes of AF, are more likely to develop post-operative AF. Post-operative AF has important implications for morbidity and mortality, and can contribute to lengthening admissions. Episodes may relate to electrolyte disturbances, hypoxia or infections, and treatment should focus on these precipitants. Otherwise, episodes should be managed as for other cases of acute-onset AF. Ideally, rhythm management should be used for AF complicating cardiac surgery.

ATRIAL FLUTTER

In atrial flutter (Figure 3.2), the electrophysiological mechanism is different from that of AF. In most patients with atrial flutter a re-entry circuit in the right atrium depolarizes at a rate of 300/min in a circular anticlockwise direction, down the lateral border of the right atrium, through an area of slowed conduction near the tricuspid valve annulus and back up the atrial septum. The normal AV node cannot conduct at this rate, and commonly 2:1 AV block occurs. The electrocardiogram shows a regular narrow complex tachycardia (in the absence of bundle branch block) at a rate of 150 bpm. This rate may be slower in a patient with impaired AV nodal function, or faster if sympathetic nervous system activation is present. Atrial activity may be visible on the ECG, seen as saw-tooth flutter waves with a rate of 300/min, best visualized in V1. The flutter waves may only be visible during a temporary increase in the degree of AV block induced by vagal manoeuvres or intravenous adenosine. It is important and useful to have documentation of the presence of flutter waves, and these procedures should be performed with

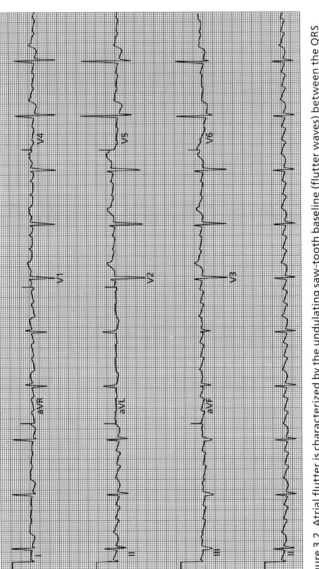

Figure 3.2 Atrial flutter is characterized by the undulating saw-tooth baseline (flutter waves) between the QRS complexes. The flutter waves are best seen in the inferior leads and lead V1. In this case the flutter rate is 250 bpm and there is 4:1 AV block.

printable ECG monitoring. Atrial flutter may degenerate into AF, or the rhythm may alternate between flutter and fibrillation.

The onset of atrial flutter may be associated with symptoms of haemodynamic compromise due to the rapid ventricular rate and loss of effective atrial mechanical activity. As with AF, there is a risk of intra-atrial clot formation in atrial flutter, leading to systemic embolization, and these patients require appropriate antithrombotic therapy as well as arrhythmia treatment. Attempts to slow the ventricular rate using drugs are often unsuccessful, and the aim of treatment should be to restore sinus rhythm. Treatment depends on the clinical circumstances:

- If the arrhythmia is associated with significant haemodynamic compromise (systolic BP <90 mmHg), or symptoms of angina, impaired conscious level or heart failure, urgent DCC is the treatment of choice.

- If the arrhythmia is well tolerated, an attempt can be made to restore sinus rhythm with drug therapy, although atrial flutter is often resistant to treatment with drugs. Class Ic antiarrhythmic drugs may terminate atrial flutter, but can also cause a poorly tolerated increase in ventricular rate (by slowing the flutter rate to less than 300/min and therefore facilitating 1:1 atrioventricular conduction at a rate greater than 150 bpm). Amiodarone has beneficial effects on atrial electrical stability, and may terminate the arrhythmia. In addition, amiodarone impairs atrioventricular conduction, and this property will help to slow the ventricular rate. We therefore recommend IV amiodarone for the treatment of atrial flutter, using the regimen detailed in Appendix A. If amiodarone is ineffective, the ventricular rate can be slowed with IV atenolol 5–10 mg. Anticoagulation and cardioversion can then be performed following the same guidelines as for AF. Overdrive pacing is an alternative treatment that is effective in restoring sinus rhythm in 70 per cent of patients. If facilities are available, a temporary pacing wire is positioned against the lateral wall of the right atrium. A burst of rapid atrial pacing at a rate of 400 bpm for several seconds will usually restore sinus rhythm. Occasionally AF will be precipitated, and this will often spontaneously revert to sinus rhythm. If it persists, it is easier to treat than atrial flutter.

- If atrial flutter persists despite 24 hours of intravenous amiodarone, or is resistant to overdrive pacing, DCC (often at very low energies) has a high success rate in restoring sinus rhythm.

Chronic drug therapy of atrial flutter has only limited efficacy. Radiofrequency ablation (with targeted lesions around the tricuspid annulus designed to interrupt the macro re-entry circuit) has much better success rates (up to 97 per cent in some cases) and is preferable for suitable patients.

ATRIOVENTRICULAR NODAL RE-ENTRY TACHYCARDIA

Background

Atrioventricular nodal re-entry is the mechanism responsible for most (70 per cent) episodes of symptomatic paroxysmal regular narrow complex tachycardia. This is a common arrhythmia, associated with recurrent attacks of palpitation throughout life, usually with an onset between 30 and 50 years of age. It is more common in women than men. In most patients there is no associated valvular, myocardial or coronary artery disease. Tachycardia onset is associated with sudden onset of rapid palpitation, which may be associated with dizziness, syncope and polyuria. The arrhythmia is usually well tolerated haemodynamically, because the heart is structurally normal. In patients with the common form of AVNRT, the AV node has two functionally and anatomically distinct pathways. These two pathways are joined into a final common pathway through the lower part of the AV node. One pathway is capable of fast conduction, and conducts electrical activity from atria to ventricles in normal sinus rhythm. The other pathway is slow conducting and is redundant during normal sinus rhythm. This slow pathway, however, has a short refractory period, and recovers its ability to conduct before the fast pathway. An appropriately timed atrial ectopic can be conducted down the slow pathway and back up the fast pathway, setting up a regular continuously reciprocating mechanism responsible for the sudden onset of a tachycardia. This re-entry in the AV node depolarizes atria and ventricles simultaneously, and resultant P waves are usually not visible because they are superimposed on the QRS complex. The ECG therefore shows a rapid regular narrow complex tachycardia (in the absence of bundle branch block) with a rate between 130 and 250 bpm and no visible P waves. (Occasionally, P waves may be visible as pseudo-R waves, particularly in lead V1 and the inferior leads.) The heart rate varies with activity of the autonomic nervous system, increasing in association with sympathetic activation (for example, standing up increases sympathetic activation, speeding up AV nodal conduction and increasing the tachycardia rate). The tachycardia can induce ST segment and T-wave changes that persist for some time after termination of the arrhythmia, but the ECG is usually normal between attacks.

Treatment

Most episodes of AVNRT can be terminated by vagal manoeuvres or intravenous drug therapy. Stimulating the vagus by a Valsalva manoeuvre, carotid sinus massage (after excluding the presence of carotid bruits) or activation of the diving reflex (by application of a cold stimulus to the face) will temporarily slow AV nodal conduction and interrupt the tachycardia circuit, terminating the arrhythmia in some patients. Some of these techniques can be used by the patient to try to terminate an attack at home, avoiding the need to attend hospital. Adenosine has a very short half-life (as short as 1.5 seconds) and no significant haemodynamic side effects. It works by transiently blocking conduction at the AV node and is very effective at terminating AVNRT. Adenosine is given as a rapid bolus at 3–6 mg into a proximal peripheral vein, often the cubital vein, and immediately flushed through with 10 mL of saline. If this fails, incremental doses of up to 18 mg can be administered. The patient should be warned that transient facial flushing, dyspnoea and chest pain are common, but last for less than 20 seconds.

Adenosine can induce bronchospasm and is contraindicated in patients with asthma or AV block. It should also be used with caution in patients with chronic obstructive pulmonary disease (COPD) because of the potential to induce or exacerbate bronchospasm. If drug-induced bronchospasm occurs, further drug administration should be avoided and, if necessary, treatment with nebulized bronchodilators commenced. Dipyridamole potentiates the effects of adenosine, and dosage should be reduced to an initial 1 mg, increasing to a maximum of 4 mg if required. Theophyllines antagonize the action of adenosine, which may render the drug ineffective in these patients.

If adenosine is contraindicated or ineffective, verapamil is an effective alternative agent, given as 5–10 mg over 30–60 seconds. Verapamil should be avoided if:

- systolic BP is <100 mmHg
- left ventricular function is known to be impaired
- QRS complex is >120 ms (three small squares)
- patient is receiving concurrent treatment with beta-blockers
- patient is known to have an anterogradely conducting accessory pathway.

If both adenosine and verapamil are contraindicated, a senior colleague should be consulted; the options would be to use a class Ic antiarrhythmic drug, or pace termination. To terminate AVNRT by pacing:

- A temporary pacing wire is placed in contact with the atrial endocardium and pacing instituted at 100 bpm. If a pacing spike occurs at an appropriate time point it will induce a critical refractory period in the circuit and terminate the arrhythmia.

- If underdrive pacing fails, the atria is paced 20 per cent faster than the tachycardia rate for 30 seconds, then the pacing abruptly terminated. This will often terminate the arrhythmia by a similar mechanism to underdrive pacing. There is a small risk of precipitating AF, which is usually short lived and reverts to sinus rhythm.

If all these measures fail, DCC can be used to restore sinus rhythm.

ACCESSORY PATHWAY TACHYCARDIAS

Background

In the normal heart the atria and ventricles become electrically isolated during fetal development. The only route by which atrial electrical activity can be conducted to the ventricles is via the AV node. Incomplete separation of the atria and ventricles during fetal development leads to the persistence of a connection that is capable of abnormally conducting electrical activity between atria and ventricles. These abnormal connections are called accessory pathways, and they can be responsible for a variety of ECG abnormalities and tachyarrhythmias. Accessory pathways are the mechanism responsible for around 20 per cent of paroxysmal regular supraventricular tachyarrhythmias. The pathways can arise in a variety of different sites around the AV rings, and connect to various areas of the ventricles or conduction system. The most common position for an accessory pathway is in the left lateral free wall of the heart. Less commonly, pathways can be situated close to the septum, in the right free wall, or, rarely, can be multiple. The appearance of the surface ECG and the type of arrhythmias that occur depend on the precise anatomy and conduction characteristics of the accessory pathway. Accessory pathway tachycardias are more common in males than females. The commonest arrhythmia in these patients arises when electrical activity repeatedly circulates between the atria and ventricles via the AV node and accessory pathway, producing an atrioventricular re-entry tachycardia (AVRT). Atrial fibrillation is a less common but potentially dangerous arrhythmia (if AF occurs in a patient with a pathway that is capable of rapid anterograde conduction from atria to ventricles, rapid activation of the ventricles can result in VF and sudden cardiac death).

Diagnosis from the ECG during sinus rhythm

In many patients with an accessory pathway, the resting ECG will be abnormal. If the pathway is capable of anterograde conduction from atria to ventricles, initial slow ventricular activation will occur via the pathway during normal sinus rhythm. This produces a short PR interval and delta wave (Figure 3.3). This type of accessory pathway is present in up to 3 per 1000 of the population (although many of these patients never have symptoms). The occurrence of arrhythmias in association with this type of pathway and abnormal ECG is termed WPW syndrome. The common left-sided pathways produce a predominantly positive QRS complex in V1. The less common right-sided pathways produce a predominantly negative QRS complex in V1. In some patients the accessory pathway is only capable of retrograde conduction from ventricles to atria. In these patients ventricular activation occurs normally via the AV node, there is no pre-excitation, and the surface ECG during sinus rhythm is completely normal. This 'concealed' accessory pathway is, however, still capable of conducting retrogradely, thereby participating in the re-entry circuit of an AVRT. The presence of a concealed accessory pathway is occasionally suggested by the characteristics of the ECG during tachycardia, indicating AV re-entry as a possible tachycardia mechanism. In most cases, however, it is difficult to distinguish AVRT from AVNRT based on the tachycardia ECG.

Atrioventricular re-entry tachycardia

Because the AV node and accessory pathway have different refractory periods, an appropriately timed ectopic can initiate a repetitive cycle of depolarization involving the AV node and accessory pathway. In the common type of AVRT, electrical activity passes to the ventricles via the AV node, then back via the accessory pathway to depolarize the atria and reinitiate the cycle (orthodromic tachycardia). Since ventricular depolarization occurs via the normal conduction system, the ECG will show a rapid regular narrow complex tachycardia (with no pre-excitation). Since atrial depolarization occurs after ventricular depolarization, an inverted P wave may be visible within the ST-T wave segments, roughly halfway between QRS complexes. Rarely, activation passes from atria to ventricles via an antegradely conducting pathway, then back to the atria via the AV node. Since ventricular depolarization is initiated via the pathway, the tachycardia will have a broad QRS morphology (antidromic

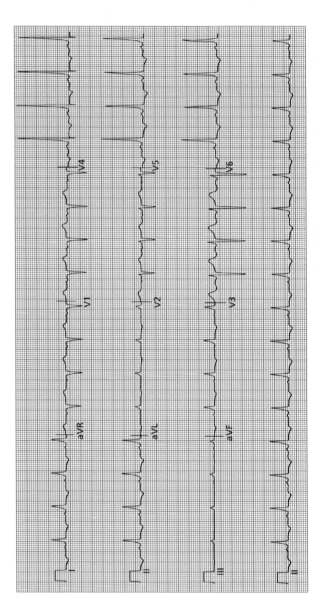

Figure 3.3 Wolff–Parkinson–White syndrome. A short PR interval and delta waves indicate the presence of an accessory pathway.

tachycardia). This type of rare AVRT is difficult to differentiate from ventricular tachycardia (VT) without the aid of an electrophysiological study (EPS).

Patients presenting with AVRT are generally similar to those with AVNRT (relatively young, no structural heart disease apparent), although AVRT is less likely to present in middle age than AVNRT.

Atrial fibrillation

AF is less common in patients with accessory pathways, but can be life threatening. The atria depolarize rapidly (350–600 impulses per minute) during AF. In a normal individual, the AV node protects the ventricles from this rapid erratic electrical activity. If AF occurs in a patient with an accessory pathway that is capable of rapid anterograde conduction, rapid atrial electrical activity can be conducted directly to the ventricles, resulting in a very fast ventricular response that can lead to haemodynamic collapse, or degenerate to VF. The ECG will show an irregularly irregular rhythm with a variable QRS morphology (due to most complexes being conducted via the pathway, leading to a broad QRS morphology, with a minority conducted via the AV node leading to a narrow QRS morphology).

Treatment

In patients with WPW sydrome who present with the common form of narrow complex orthodromic tachycardia and who are not haemodynamically compromised, initial drug therapy is appropriate. As a general principle, drugs that predominantly block AV nodal conduction should be avoided in patients known to have an accessory pathway. In certain circumstances, AV nodal blocking drugs can cause tachycardia acceleration (for instance, in patients with AF and a pathway capable of rapid anterograde conduction). It is therefore preferable to use a drug that acts predominantly to slow accessory pathway conduction. Intravenous flecainide 2 mg/kg (maximum 150 mg) has a good safety profile in a patient with an accessory pathway, and will terminate more than 80 per cent of episodes. If flecainide fails, consult a senior colleague before administering another drug. If the patient is haemodynamically compromised with the tachycardia, DCC is the treatment of choice.

When AF occurs in a patient with a pathway capable of rapid anterograde conduction, the ventricular rate can exceed 250 bpm. These rapid ventricular rates are often associated with haemodynamic compromise or heart failure, and urgent DC cardioversion is required. If the AF is slower and well tolerated, a drug that slows accessory pathway conduction (such as flecainide 2 mg/kg IV) can be used to slow the ventricular rate and restore sinus rhythm.

Because of the inherent risk of sudden death, all patients with an accessory pathway should be reviewed by an electrophysiologist to plan an optimal investigation and treatment strategy. The most dangerous pathways are those that are capable of rapid antegrade conduction from atria to ventricles. Concealed pathways and pathways that show intermittent pre-excitation or pre-excitation that disappears with exercise are unlikely to be capable of rapid antegrade conduction, but electrophysiological characterization of the conduction characteristics of the pathway is more reliable than inspection of the surface ECG. Ablation is highly successful and low risk, and should be considered for all patients with an accessory pathway (the risks of long-term antiarrhythmic drug therapy are probably greater than the procedure-related risks of EPS and ablation).

ATRIAL TACHYCARDIA

Atrial tachycardia is relatively rare. Unifocal atrial tachycardia arises from a single repetitively discharging area of micro re-entry or enhanced automaticity. During the arrhythmia the ECG will usually show a regular narrow complex tachycardia with a rate of 120–240 bpm (Figure 3.4). Each QRS complex will be preceded by a morphologically abnormal P wave, usually best seen in V1. An upright P wave in V1 indicates the tachycardia is due to a left atrial focus, a positive P wave in AVL indicates a right atrial origin. The arrhythmia can arise in patients with structural heart disease leading to atrial dilatation or dysfunction, particularly in patients with cardiorespiratory co-morbidities, but commonly no cause is found. Atrial tachycardia is often resistant to drug therapy. Nodal blocking drugs will not terminate the arrhythmia, but may slow the ventricular rate. Antiarrhythmic drugs that stabilize atrial electrical activity (such as sotalol, flecainide and amiodarone) may terminate the arrhythmia. If drug therapy fails, overdrive pacing or cardioversion should be considered. Unifocal atrial tachycardias are readily treated by ablation in suitable patients who have recurrent symptoms.

Unifocal atrial tachycardia may arise as a complication of digoxin toxicity. In this case, digoxin induces a variable degree of atrioventricular block as well as triggering the discharge of an atrial

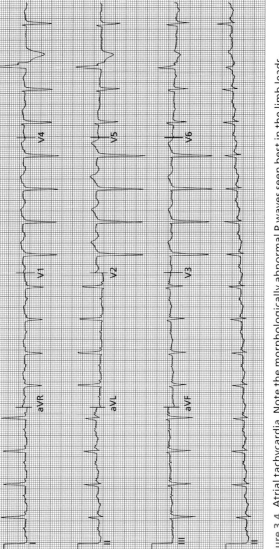

Figure 3.4 Atrial tachycardia. Note the morphologically abnormal P waves seen best in the limb leads.

ectopic focus. The atrial rate is generally 150–200 bpm, and the degree of atrioventricular block may fluctuate, producing an irregular ventricular rhythm. When atrial tachycardia with variable block complicates digoxin therapy:

- further digoxin therapy should be withheld until the arrhythmia resolves
- beta-blockers should be given (if necessary) to slow the ventricular rate
- potassium should be maintained above 4.0 mmol/L
- Digibind (see Chapter 8) should be considered.

DCC should be avoided, as it may induce intractable arrhythmias in a patient with digoxin toxicity.

Multifocal atrial tachycardia most commonly arises as a complication of respiratory disease in acutely ill elderly patients, and is characterized by multiple atrial foci producing constant variation in the P-wave morphology and a variable atrial rate (Figure 3.5). Therapy consists of ensuring that the potassium level is adequate, treating the underlying respiratory problem, and using AV nodal blocking drugs to control the ventricular rate.

VENTRICULAR ARRHYTHMIAS

Background

A tachycardia with broad QRS complexes can be due to:

- VT
- supraventricular tachycardia in a patient with pre-existing or rate-related bundle branch block
- supraventricular tachycardia in a patient with an accessory pathway that is capable of anterograde conduction.

A series of clinical and ECG guidelines can be used to determine the site of tachycardia origin. The patient's general clinical state is no guide to the site of tachycardia origin. The degree of haemodynamic compromise that occurs depends on the ventricular rate and left ventricular function. A rapid supraventricular tachycardia in a patient with left ventricular dysfunction may cause major haemodynamic collapse, whilst a slow VT may be well tolerated in a patient with good left ventricular function. If the patient is not severely compromised, clinical assessment, a 12-lead ECG or the use of IV adenosine helps to

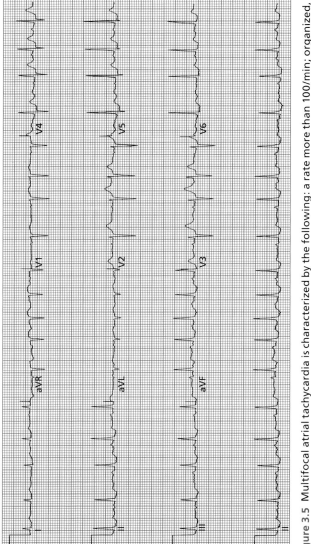

Figure 3.5 Multifocal atrial tachycardia is characterized by the following: a rate more than 100/min; organized, discrete non-sinus P waves with at least three different forms in the same ECG lead; isoelectric baseline between P waves; and irregular PP, PR and RR intervals. In patients with heart rates less than 100/min, the term multifocal atrial rhythm is used.

identify the site of origin of a broad complex tachycardia. The useful features are:

- A totally irregular broad complex tachycardia is likely to be AF with bundle branch block or an accessory pathway.

- Capture or fusion beats, independent P waves that are dissociated from ventricular activity or clinical evidence of AV dissociation (cannon waves or variable intensity S1) confirm that the tachycardia is VT.

- A broad QRS (>140 ms), marked axis deviation, ventricular concordance, a deep S wave in V6 or an RSr pattern in V1 suggest a ventricular origin (Figure 3.6).

- If an IV adenosine bolus has no effect on the tachycardia, it is probably VT. If the arrhythmia terminates, it is probably of supraventricular origin. The transient period of AV block associated with adenosine administration may allow visualization of atrial fibrillation, flutter or tachycardia activity.

It is important to remember that the vast majority of broad complex tachycardias are due to VT, particularly if the patient is known to have structural heart disease. Intravenous verapamil should never be given to a patient with a broad complex tachycardia as it may cause severe and intractable haemodynamic depression if the tachycardia is VT. If doubt as to the diagnosis remains after clinical assessment, inspection of the ECG and administration of adenosine, then the arrhythmia should be treated as VT.

Monomorphic VT

The commonest cause of monomorphic VT is ischaemic heart disease. Monomorphic VT occurring early in the course of an ACS is usually due to enhanced automaticity in an infarcting segment of myocardium. Monomorphic VT occurring late after an ACS is usually associated with re-entry in scar tissue. Less common causes include cardiomyopathy, myocarditis, arrhythmogenic right ventricular dysplasia, valvular heart disease, or scarring associated with cardiac surgery. Occasionally, monomorphic VT can arise in an entirely normal heart. The occurrence of monomorphic VT with a left bundle and right axis configuration in a patient with a normal heart indicates that the arrhythmia is arising from the right ventricular outflow tract. A relatively narrow QRS duration suggests that the origin of the tachycardia lies close to the bundle of His (fascicular VT). Both

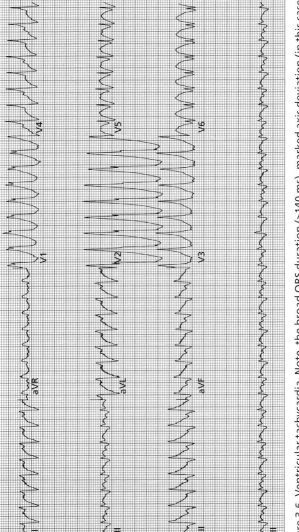

Figure 3.6 Ventricular tachycardia. Note, the broad QRS duration (>140 ms), marked axis deviation (in this case right axis deviation), RSr pattern in lead V1, deep S in lead V5 and V6, AV dissociation (best seen in lead II) and a fusion beat (nineteenth QRS complex on the rhythm strip).

these tachycardias can be terminated by adenosine and are amenable to radiofrequency ablation. If the resting ECG shows T-wave inversion in V1–V3 and there is a family history of palpitations or sudden death, arrhythmogenic right ventricular dysplasia is a possibility. If the arrhythmia is exercise induced in a structurally normal heart, right ventricular outflow tachycardia is a possibility. If there is evidence of conduction tissue disease then bundle branch re-entry tachycardia should be considered.

Monomorphic VT consists of a rapid succession of ventricular ectopic beats occurring at a rate >120 bpm. The rhythm will be predominantly regular and each successive ventricular complex will have a uniform appearance. The regularity and morphology of the tachycardia may be intermittently altered by the occurrence of capture of fusion beats. Monomorphic VT that lasts for less than 30 seconds is defined as non-sustained. A right bundle branch block configuration indicates a left ventricular origin for the tachycardia, whilst a left bundle branch block configuration indicates a right ventricular origin. Treatment of sustained monomorphic VT is detailed in Chapter 1. If the monomorphic VT is not clearly related to an ACS, there is a high risk of recurrence, and expert investigation is required to determine the underlying cause. The investigations to consider are:

- coronary angiography to evaluate the presence and extent of coronary artery disease in patients with ischaemic heart disease
- cardiac imaging with echocardiography or MRI to evaluate cardiac structure and function in patients with cardiomyopathy
- stress testing to look for exercise-induced ischaemia or VT.

If an identifiable precipitating factor such as cardiac ischaemia can be identified, this should be treated before using antiarrhythmic drugs. If there is no clear treatable factor, drug therapy or implantation of an implantable cardioverter defibrillator (ICD) should be considered. An ICD is preferable if the VT was associated with cardiac arrest, major haemodynamic compromise, the patient has an ejection fraction of <35 per cent or an abnormality such as cardiomyopathy is present. If the patient is not suitable for ICD implantation, drug therapy is an inferior alternative. The most effective drugs to prevent recurrence of VT are beta-blockers, sotalol and amiodarone.

Polymorphic VT
Polymorphic VT is characterized by repeated progressive changes in QRS morphology and orientation, producing an appearance of twisting

around the baseline (Figure 3.7). Polymorphic VT in the absence of QT prolongation is mainly associated with ACS, and is dealt with in Chapter 1. Polymorphic VT occurring in association with QT prolongation is termed Torsade de Pointes tachycardia. This type of VT occurs when abnormal ventricular repolarization with resultant QT prolongation occurs due to bradycardia, hypokalaemia, hypomagnesaemia or drugs. The common drugs associated with QT prolongation are antiarrhythmics, antibiotics, antihistamines and antipsychotics. Rarely, QT prolongation may be congenital, when it is due to inherited or sporadic genetic defects of myocyte potassium and sodium channels. Treatment consists of:

- withdrawal of any implicated drugs
- treatment of sustained episodes with DCC if associated with haemodynamic collapse
- pacing at 100 bpm to shorten the QT interval
- giving IV magnesium 8 mmol stat then 2.5 mmol/h infusion for 24 hours.

In patients with congenital QT prolongation, beta-blockade (excluding sotalol), sympathectomy or an ICD may be required.

Ventricular fibrillation

The commonest cause of VF is ischaemic heart disease, and it is responsible for 90 per cent of deaths related to ACS. The emergency management of VF is dealt with in Chapters 1 and 2. If VF occurs in the absence of evidence of an ACS, careful investigation is required as described for VT. All patients who survive an episode of VF not associated with ACS should be considered for an ICD, as this is prognostically more effective than drug therapy.

BRADYARRHYTHMIAS

Background

Bradyarrhythmias arising as a complication of ACS (particularly inferior STEMI) are dealt with in Chapter 1. Bradyarrhythmias that are not related to an ACS are most commonly due to idiopathic fibrosis of the conduction system (which is more common in the elderly), although a wide range of other cardiac conditions can occasionally be responsible. These bradyarrhythmias may present with important symptoms that require urgent treatment.

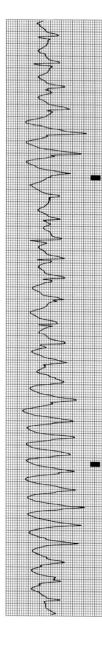

Figure 3.7 Polymorphic VT. Note the frequent changes in QRS complex morphology.

Atrioventricular block

First degree heart block (prolongation of the PR interval to >200 msec) signifies slow conduction of electrical activity from atria to ventricles (Figure 3.8). First degree block does not cause symptoms, and can occur in young people in association with high vagal tone. In older individuals it may indicate the presence of underlying fibrosis in the conduction system with a risk of progression to higher grade AV block. In second degree block there is intermittent failure of conduction of atrial impulses to the ventricles, manifest as a P wave not followed by a QRS complex. In Mobitz type 1 (Wenckebach) second degree AV block, a progressive increase in impaired conduction in the AV node occurs with each successive sinus beat. This leads to a progressive prolongation in the PR interval until an atrial impulse fails to be conducted, resulting in a dropped beat. After the dropped beat, AV conduction recovers and the sequence is repeated. Mobitz type 1 block can be a benign phenomenon occurring in normal individuals with high vagal tone, particularly during sleep. In the absence of high vagal tone in a younger individual, Mobitz type 1 block is associated with a significant risk of progression to high degree AV block with symptoms. In Mobitz type 2 second degree AV block, impaired conduction in the bundle of His or bundle branches leads to intermittent failure of conduction of atrial impulses to the ventricles without preceding lengthening of the PR interval. These patients often have associated bundle branch block and axis deviation (bifascicular block), occasionally with associated PR interval prolongation, reflecting extensive disease in the bundle of His. Patients with Mobitz type 2 block have extensive conduction system disease and are at increased risk of Stokes–Adams attacks, slow ventricular rates and sudden death. Complete heart block occurs when there is total failure of conduction of electrical activity from atria to ventricles (Figure 3.9). Complete heart block can be due to disease at nodal or bundle of His level. If the block is at nodal level, the escape rhythm that results will be narrow complex, stable and usually fast enough to support an adequate circulation. In patients with extensive disease in the bundle of His, the subsidiary pacemaker will be low in the conduction system, producing a slow, unreliable broad complex escape rhythm, with an increased risk of major symptoms.

Sino-atrial node disease

When fibrosis predominantly affects the sinus node and atria, sino-atrial node (SAN) disease (or sick sinus syndrome) occurs. This is characterized

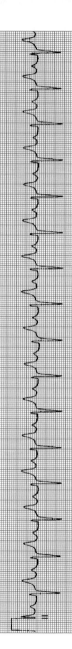

Figure 3.8 First degree AV block characterized by a PR interval of >200 msec.

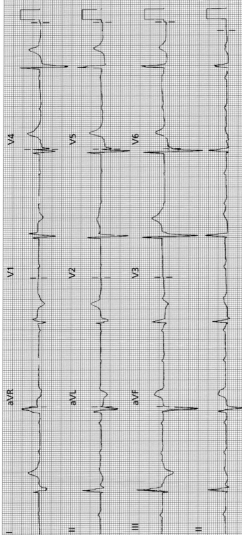

Figure 3.9 Complete heart block. There is complete AV dissociation with the P waves and QRS complexes occurring without any relation to each other. Note the constantly changing PR intervals.

by a variety of often intermittent tachy- or bradyarrhythmias. The common rhythm disturbances are:

- sinus bradycardia
- sinus arrest
- atrial flutter or fibrillation.

In up to one-third of these patients the fibrotic process extends into the AV node and heart block coexists.

Clinical features and management

The electrocardiographic features of heart block are discussed in Chapter 1. In SAN disease the ECG shows sinus bradycardia, sinus arrest, atrial fibrillation or flutter and sometimes AV block (these features may only be evident with prolonged rhythm monitoring). First degree and Mobitz type 1 AV block do not cause symptoms. If the conduction disturbance is not clearly associated with high vagal tone, close monitoring is required as higher grade AV block may develop. In patients with bifascicular block, there is a small risk of progression to complete heart block, but pacing in the absence of symptoms is not required. If general anaesthesia is required for non-cardiac surgery in a patient with bifascicular block and prolongation of the PR interval (trifasicular block), many authorities recommend prophylactic temporary pacing to guard against sudden complete heart block.

In Mobitz type 2 and complete heart block a slow ventricular rate may cause tiredness, dyspnoea or heart failure. If the escape rhythm is unreliable or intermittently fails, syncope or sudden death may occur. Patients with SAN disease have bradyarrhythmia-related syncope or dizziness which may be associated with palpitations due to tachyarrhythmias.

Patients who present with symptomatic bradyarrhythmias due to chronic conduction system disease may require short-term support to maintain an adequate heart rate. If there is a history of dizziness or syncope associated with a ventricular rate of <40 bpm (particularly if the escape rhythm is broad complex), or pauses of >3 seconds, then treatment is required. The options are:

- to commence an isoprenaline infusion (Appendix A) to increase the ventricular rate
- to apply an external pacing system for temporary rate support
- to insert a temporary pacing wire.

The complication rate for temporary pacing is high for inexperienced operators. The first two options are preferable in the absence of an appropriately skilled operator, and are discussed in more detail in Chapter 2. If temporary pacing is used, the femoral vein provides a good access site that minimizes the risk of access site complications and also reduces the amount of pacing lead manipulation required. If the patient has a rate of >40 bpm with a narrow complex escape rhythm and no long pauses, it is appropriate to monitor the rhythm in a coronary care unit environment, avoiding rhythm support initially. All patients with symptomatic chronic bradyarrhythmias should be considered for permanent pacing.

KEY POINTS

- Selecting the best treatment depends on the mechanism and effect of an arrhythmia.

- QRS duration is not a totally reliable guide to the site of origin of an arrhythmia.

- Antiarrhythmic drug therapy has many limitations (due to poor efficacy and side effects).

- AF is common – treatment depends on the duration of the arrhythmia and its haemodynamic effects. Atrial flutter is relatively uncommon, and is treated in a similar fashion to AF.

- The commonest cause of recurrent narrow complex tachycardia is AV nodal re-entry (which usually can be terminated by adenosine).

- Accessory pathways are not always associated with an abnormal resting ECG. The commonest associated arrhythmia is a regular narrow complex tachycardia with P waves visible between QRS complexes; AF is rare but can be dangerous.

- A broad complex tachycardia can be due to VT, bundle branch block or an accessory pathway. Most of these tachycardias are VT.

- Many bradyarrhythmias are well tolerated and emergency pacing should be avoided if possible.

KEY REFERENCES

Blaauw Y, Crijns HJGM. Treatment of atrial fibrillation. *Heart* 2008; **94**: 1342–9.
Brugada P, Brugada J, Mont L, Smeets J, Andries EW. A new approach to the differential diagnosis of a regular tachycardia with a wide QRS complex. *Circulation* 1991; **83**: 1649–59.

Camm AJ, Garratt CJ. Adenosine and supraventricular tachycardia. *N Engl J Med* 1991; **325**: 1621–9.

DaCosta D, Brady WJ, Edhouse J. ABC of clinical electrocardiography. Bradycardias and atrioventricular conduction block. *BMJ* 2002; **324**: 535–8.

Dancy M, Ward D. Diagnosis of ventricular tachycardia: a clinical algorithm. *BMJ* 1989; **291**: 1036–8.

Edhouse J, Morris F. ABC of clinical electrocardiography. Broad complex tachycardia – Part I. *BMJ* 2002; **324**: 719–22.

Edhouse J, Morris F. ABC of clinical electrocardiography. Broad complex tachycardia – Part II. *BMJ* 2002; **324**: 776–9.

Esberger D, Jones S, Morris F. ABC of clinical electrocardiography: junctional tachycardias. *BMJ* 2002; **324**: 662–5.

Fox DJ, Tischenko A, Krahn AD, et al. Supraventricular tachycardia: diagnosis and management. *Mayo Clin Proc* 2008; **83**: 1400–11.

Ganz LI, Friedman PL. Supraventricular tachycardia. *N Engl J Med* 1995; **332**: 162–73.

Goodacre S, Irons R. ABC of clinical electrocardiography: atrial arrhythmias. *BMJ* 2002; **324**: 594–7.

Julian DG. The amiodarone trials. *Eur Heart J* 1997; **18**: 1361–3.

Kowey PR, Marinchak RA, Rials SJ, Filart RA. Intravenous amiodarone. *J Am Coll Cardiol* 1997; **29**: 1190–8.

Levy S, Ricard P. Using the right drug: a treatment algorithm for regular supraventricular tachycardias. *Eur Heart J* 1997; **18**(Suppl C): C27–C32.

Murphy JJ. Problems with temporary cardiac pacing. *BMJ* 2001; **323**: 527.

Obel OA, Camm AJ. Supraventricular tachycardia: ECG and anatomy. *Eur Heart J* 1997; **18**(Suppl C): C2–C11.

Peters NS, Schilling RJ, Kanagaratnam P, Markides V. Atrial fibrillation: strategies to control, combat, and cure. *Lancet* 2002; **359**: 593–603.

Pye M, Camm AJ. Supraventricular tachycardia: a comprehensive review of the diagnosis and management of supraventricular tachycardia. *Hosp Update* 1996; **22**: 226–37.

Rankin AC, Cobbe SM. Broad-complex tachycardias. *Prescribers J* 1993; **33**: 138–46.

Roden DM. Risks and benefits of antiarrhythmic therapy. *N Engl J Med* 1994; **331**: 785–91.

Van Gelder IC, Hagens VE, Bosker HA, et al. A comparison of rate control and rhythm control in patients with recurrent persistent atrial fibrillation. *N Engl J Med* 2002; **347**: 1834–40.

Wellens HJJ. The value of the ECG in the diagnosis of supraventricular tachycardias. *Eur Heart J* 1996; **17**(Suppl C): 10–20.

Wellens HJJ. Ventricular tachycardia: diagnosis of broad QRS complex tachycardia. *Heart* 2001; **86**: 579–85.

Wyse DG, Waldo AL, DiMarco JP, et al. A comparison of rate control and rhythm control in patients with atrial fibrillation. *N Engl J Med* 2002; **347**: 1825–33.

HYPERTENSIVE EMERGENCIES

BACKGROUND

Epidemiology

In a small proportion of patients with hypertension, an accelerated phase of the disease may develop into malignant hypertension. This presents clinically as a hypertensive emergency with marked elevation of blood pressure accompanied by end-organ damage. The frequency of hypertensive emergencies is declining due to widespread early treatment of less severe hypertension, with contemporary incidence rates of around 1 per cent in hypertensive subjects. A hypertensive crisis is commonest in the young black male population.

This accelerated phase may present us a medical emergency in which the blood pressure should be reduced immediately to avoid irreversible target organ damage. The urgent need for blood pressure control is most acute where life-threatening complications such as an aortic dissection or encephalopathy occur. Any hypertensive condition can develop into a crisis, although it is commoner in secondary forms of the disease such as with phaeochromocytoma and in renovascular hypertension. Prior to the introduction of effective antihypertensive therapy, less than 25 per cent of patients with malignant hypertension survived 1 year, with a 1 per cent 5-year survival. In the current era with renal dialysis support, 1- and 5-year survival is 90 per cent and 80 per cent, respectively. In severe hypertension, early death is usually due to stroke or acute renal failure. In the longer term, coronary artery disease becomes the commonest cause of death.

Hypertensive emergencies are most common in patients with long-standing, poorly controlled chronic hypertension, often following an abrupt cessation in antihypertensive therapy. In these patients, chronic vascular changes provide a degree of protection to the end organs. In previously normotensive patients who develop an acute rise in blood pressure (for example, as a complication of acute renal failure or pregnancy) there are no chronic vascular adaptive changes to limit the adverse effects of the hypertension, and severe end-organ damage can occur at lower pressures.

Pathophysiology

Any cause of hypertension can lead to a hypertensive emergency (Table 4.1). The likelihood of severe adverse effects is highest in patients who develop a rapid increase in systemic blood pressure: the vascular adaptation to chronic hypertension reduces the likelihood of end-organ damage, with the corollary that in the absence of pre-existing hypertension, a hypertensive emergency can occur at a lower pressure. A hypertensive emergency occurs when sustained diastolic blood pressure is above 130 mmHg leading to a risk of end-organ damage.

The exact initiating step in a hypertensive crisis is not well understood. There is a cascade of physiological decompensation initiated by a critical degree of hypertension, which occurs both systemically and locally in vascular beds. An increase in vasoreactivity occurs. The renin-angiotensin-aldosterone system is crucial in the development of this hyper-reactivity. Angiotensin II is a potent vasoconstrictor and also has direct cytotoxic effects on endothelium through activation of gene expression or pro-inflammatory cytokines such as interleukin-6 (IL-6) and the transcription factor, NF-κb. Inhibition of tissue angiotensin converting enzyme (ACE) can prevent malignant hypertension in transgenic mice. Systemically, there is activation of the sympathetic nervous system, the renin-angiotensin-aldosterone system and increased release of antidiuretic hormone. This leads to systemic vasoconstriction and a rise in vascular resistance, as well as an increase in circulating blood volume. Paradoxically, the baroreceptor response to this is overwhelmed with a further increase in circulating vasopressor hormones. Locally, free radical production and endothelin release is associated with further endothelial dysfunction, growth factor release and vascular smooth muscle cell proliferation diminishing local vascular autoregulation. Progressive endothelial dysfunction through pro-inflammatory cytokines with up-regulation of endothelial adhesion molecules (such as E- and P-selectin) promotes

Table 4.1 Causes of hypertensive emergencies

Essential hypertension

Renal parenchymal disease

- acute glomerulonephritis
- renal vasculitis
- haemolytic uraemic syndrome
- thrombotic thrombocytopenic purpura

Renovascular disease

Pregnancy

- eclampsia

Endocrine disease

- phaeochromocytoma
- hypheradrenalism (Cushing's syndrome)
- renin-secreting tumours

Drugs

- cocaine abuse
- sympathomimetic abuse
- erythropoietin in haemodialysis patients
- cyclosporin A
- interactions with monoamine oxidase inhibitors (tyramine ingestion)

Autonomic hyper-reactivity

- Guillain–Barré syndrome
- acute intermittent porphyria

Neurological disease

- head injury
- cerebrovascular accident
- brain tumours

local inflammation. An increase in vascular permeability and activation of the coagulation cascade is the consequence of this, promoting further vasoconstriction. The end result of these adverse changes in neuroendocrine and vascular function is an acute rise in blood pressure, with diastolic pressures consistently exceeding 130 mmHg. The severe elevation in blood pressure leads to widespread fibrinoid necrosis in small arteries and arterioles. Thrombotic occlusion of these damaged vessels is common, leading to infarction in end organs. These damaged vessels also exhibit increased permeability leading to tissue oedema.

There are several important vascular beds which are at risk during a hypertensive emergency:

- **Cerebrovascular:** hypertensive encephalopathy is an acute medical emergency characterized by headache, irritability, an altered conscious level, seizures and coma. The acute diffuse neurological effects of malignant hypertension are reversed by prompt reduction in the blood pressure. Other potential complications of a hypertensive crisis are intracerebral or subarachnoid haemorrhage, and thrombotic infarction in individuals with predisposing atherosclerotic cerebrovascular disease.

- **Cardiovascular:** acute left ventricular failure (LVF) or an acute coronary syndrome may occur due to the inability of a stiffened, hypertrophied left ventricle to cope with a sudden rise in systemic vascular resistance. Acute aortic dissection is a potential complication of a hypertensive crisis, particularly in patients with cystic medial necrosis of the thoracic aorta.

- **Renal:** haematuria and progressive renal failure can occur.

The commonest clinical manifestations are of cerebral infarction (25 per cent), pulmonary oedema (23 per cent), encephalopathy (16 per cent) and congestive cardiac failure (12 per cent).

Clinical features

Malignant hypertension is associated with a persistent diastolic pressure of greater that 130 mmHg. Other diagnostic clinical features of malignant hypertensive crisis include:

- hypertensive retinopathy
  - haemorrhage, exudates and papilloedema (grades 3 and 4 hypertensive retinopathy)

- hypertensive encephalopathy
  - headache, confusion, altered consciousness, leading to seizure activity and coma

- acute renal failure
  - protein and red blood cells noted on urinalysis
  - hypokalaemia from secondary hyperaldosteronism
  - oliguria may ensue
- microangiopathic haemolytic anaemia

When any of these features are present, immediate treatment to lower blood pressure is required.

Miscellaneous situations

In certain other hypertensive crises, an immediate reduction in blood pressure is required:

- phaeochromocytoma
- food or drug interactions with monoamine oxidase inhibitors
- head injury
- post-operative bleeding
- severe, uncontrollable epistaxis

There are other clinical situations where a quick rather than immediate reduction of blood pressure is required:

- malignant hypertension with no end-organ compromise
- rebound hypertension after drug withdrawal
- severe hypertension post-surgery
- severe widespread burn injury

CLINICAL EVALUATION

History

An accurate history of the duration and severity of any pre-existing hypertension must be established. It is equally important to establish the presence of end-organ damage, such as hypertensive renal disease and cerebrovascular disease. Symptoms of target organ injury may be present:

- anterior chest pain: myocardial ischaemia, acute aortic dissection;
- posterior chest pain: aortic dissection;
- dyspnoea: acute pulmonary oedema, acute heart failure;
- altered consciousness/seizures: encephalopathy.

It is important to take a complete drug history to establish both any pre-existing therapy and the possibility of recent drug withdrawal or non-compliance. The recreational abuse of cocaine or other sympathomimetic drugs should be considered.

Physical examination

- Blood pressure measurement – in both arms, erect and supine
- Cardiovascular examination – presence of heart failure (raised jugular venous pressure (JVP), third heart sound, pulmonary crepitations)
- Neurological examination – conscious level, visual fields, focal pyramidal signs
- Fundoscopy – new haemorrhages, exudates and papilloedema indicate a hypertensive emergency.

Investigations

Initial investigations:

- Biochemistry – urea, creatinine and electrolytes
- Haemotology – full blood count, including a blood film for evidence of haemolysis
- 12-lead ECG – to exclude/confirm ischaemia, to indicate left ventricular hypertrophy
- Chest x-ray – look for evidence of heart failure or dissection
- Urinalysis – red blood cells, protein.

Additional investigations should include:

- echocardiography
- renal ultrasound scan
- computed tomography of thorax and abdomen, and
- magnetic resonance renovascular and neuro-imaging (see below).

MANAGEMENT

The treatment of a hypertensive crisis is based on consensus rather than on randomized controlled trials. The first principle of care is that a hypertensive emergency patient is managed in a high-dependency environment with withdrawal of any potential treatments that may be exacerbating the situation. This allows for accurate and continuous blood pressure monitoring with an arterial line. Treatment should be initiated by the intravenous route and titrated against the antihypertensive response. Combination therapy is preferred to achieve an additive effect and may be tailored towards any compromise in a particular end organ. In aortic dissection, a combination of intravenous beta-blockade (labetalol, which is a mixed alpha- and beta-blocker) given first followed by sodium nitroprusside is the preferred therapy. In the presence of myocardial ischaemia, intravenous glyceryl trinitrate with beta-blockade gives maximum anti-ischaemic effect, albeit with a diminishing antihypertensive effect over time. In aortic dissection, a relatively rapid reduction in systolic blood pressure (SBP) to <110 mmHg should be aimed for. In hypertensive encephalopathy, centrally acting drugs should be avoided, and the aim should be to reduce mean arterial pressure (MAP) by 25 per cent over 8 hours. Where cerebral infarction has occurred, rapid reductions in blood pressure should be avoided to avoid cerebral hypoperfusion in the context of impaired autoregulation, and care must be taken if fibrinolytic therapy is being considered. In cases of intracerebral haemorrhage, blood pressure lowering should also be performed gradually. When associated with signs of increased intracranial pressure (ICP), MAP should be maintained just below 130 mmHg (or SBP <180 mmHg) for the first 24 hours. For those without increased ICP, a MAP <110 mmHg (or SBP <160 mmHg) should be maintained for the first 24 hours.

SPECIFIC DRUG THERAPY

Sodium nitroprusside

This short-acting arterial and venous dilator is first-line therapy for a hypertensive emergency. It has an immediate effect and its dose may be titrated against its efficacy. This will allow the simultaneous administration of oral antihypertensive agents, facilitating discontinuation of the nitroprusside infusion before the risk of thiocyanate toxicity. It is given in a dose of 0.25–10 µg/kg/min.

Labetalol

This mixed alpha- and beta-adrenergic blocker is the other mainstay of therapy in a hypertensive emergency. Although its beta-blocking effect is weaker than conventional beta-blockers, it can be given in bolus form at a dose of 20–80 mg in addition to an intravenous infusion of 2 mg/min.

ACE inhibition

These drugs are effective in lowering blood pressure within 15 minutes of an intravenous bolus such as enalaprilat (1.25–5 mg), with an effect lasting at least 4 hours. However, precipitous falls may occur in patients with hypovolaemia or significant renovascular disease. In accelerated hypertension, a pressure-induced natriuresis may occur, leading to the confounding physiological situation of hypovolaemia in the setting of hypertension.

Fenoldopam

This drug is approved for use in hypertensive emergencies. It is a peripheral dopamine-1 receptor agonist, which peripherally vasodilates with an additional potent vasodilating effect on renal arteries. It has a quick onset (5 minutes) and is used at a dose of 0.1–0.6 µg/kg/min. In one study compared with sodium nitroprusside, fenoldopam improved renal dysfunction in severely hypertensive patients with renal impairment.

Glyceryl trinitrate

Intravenous GTN (5–100 µg/min) is of particular use where significant coronary artery disease coexists with a hypertensive emergency. Although not a potent therapy for hypertension itself, the restoration of the imbalance between myocardial demand and supply through reduction in intramyocardial wall tension, preload reduction and improved collateral blood supply is of benefit, particularly when used in conjunction with beta-blockade. Like sodium nitroprusside, afterload reduction is of benefit in the presence of LVF.

A recent systematic review of 15 randomized controlled trials was unable to find evidence that antihypertensive drugs reduced mortality or morbidity in patients with hypertensive emergencies (there were no randomized studies specifically addressing this issue). Further, there was insufficient evidence to determine which drug or drug class was most effective in reducing mortality and morbidity. Whilst there were some small differences in degree of blood pressure lowering among classes, the clinical significance was unclear. The review demonstrated evidence of blood pressure lowering efficacy for nitrates, ACE inhibitors, diuretics, alpha-adrenergic antagonists, calcium channel blockers and dopamine agonists. Nitrates (including nitroprusside) were the most studied group, making this class of drug a reasonable choice of therapy in hypertensive emergencies.

SPECIFIC HYPERTENSIVE EMERGENCIES

Hypertensive encephalopathy

There are both functional and structural processes which occur in the brain when there is an acute sustained increase in systemic blood pressure. The functional response to an excessive perfusion pressure is cerebral arteriolar vasodilatation (rather than vasoconstriction as expected) and a loss of microcirculatory autoregulation, leading to the leakage of fluid into the perivascular space and cerebral oedema. With acute endothelial injury, the structural changes in the arterioles lead to an increase in vascular permeability independent of the renin-angiotensin-aldosterone system. This leads to disruption of the blood–brain barrier, cerebral oedema and micro-haemorrhage. The normal range over which vital organs such as the brain and the heart autoregulate blood flow in the face of varying perfusion pressure (MAP) is between 60 and 120 mmHg. In patients with pre-existing hypertension, this autoregulatory range is increased to between 110 and 180 mmHg through an increase in the intimal area of the larger resistive vessels (pre-arterioles) that deliver perfusion to the smaller resistive vessels (arterioles). These former vessels are influenced by the perfusion pressure and cerebral blood flow, and by myogenic tone. Conversely, in patients with no previous hypertension, signs of encephalopathy can occur at a pressure as low as 160/100 mmHg. Thus, the clinical response is largely dependent on whether the patient develops the hypertensive crisis in the context of a previously normal blood pressure.

Hypertensive encephalopathy is characterized by the acute onset of lethargy, confusion, headache, visual disturbance and focal or generalized seizures. If untreated, coma, cerebral haemorrhage and death may ensue. Intracerebral haemorrhage is particularly likely in thrombotic thrombocytopenic purpura and in pre-eclampsia where haemolysis occurs with acute liver injury and thrombocytopenia occurs. Magnetic resonance imaging with T_2-weighting may confirm a posterior leucoencephalopathy affecting predominantly the white matter of the parieto-occipital regions (largely bilateral). The cerebellum and brainstem may also be affected, and occasionally the cerebral cortex. The posterior cerebral predilection occurs through a reduction in sympathetic innervation accompanying the basilar artery and its branches.

Hypertensive encephalopathy is reversible, leading to the specific term hypertensive reversible posterior leucoencephalopathy syndrome (PLS). It has been described in both children and adults and may also occur in non-hypertensive situations such as through drug toxicity (cyclosporin and tacrolimus [often an acute cause of hypertension], cisplatin and interferon-α therapy), acquired immunodeficiency syndrome (AIDS), thrombotic thrombocytopenic purpura and after blood transfusion.

Although the aim of treatment is to bring the diastolic pressure down to around 100 mmHg within the first hour, it is important to be aware that patients with pre-existing hypertension and elderly patients are at particular risk of a watershed infarct with aggressive blood pressure reduction. In patients with seizure activity, anticonvulsant therapy using intravenous phenytoin or benzodiazepines should be given additionally.

Phaeochromocytoma

Phaeochromocytoma arise from sympathetic ganglia derived from the primitive neural crest with 90 per cent arising from the adrenal medulla, 10 per cent bilateral and 10 per cent malignant rather than benign. They account for up to 0.2 per cent of hypertensive patients. These 'tumours', which are essentially extreme nodular hyperplasia, may occur as part of the familial multiple endocrine neoplasia (MEN-2) syndrome. They create extreme fluctuations in systemic blood pressure with associated symptoms, although the hypertension becomes persistent in half of patients. With adrenaline as the predominant catecholamine secreted (mainly from adrenal medullary tumours), symptoms of an increased cardiac output with systolic hypertension, sinus tachycardia, sweating, flushing and apprehension occur. Noradrenaline is usually the predominant hormone (adrenal and most extra-adrenal tumours), and there is an increased peripheral vasoconstriction with diastolic as well as systolic hypertension with less tachycardia or palpitations. In 45 per cent, the hypertension is paroxysmal, and often occurs in response to anaesthesia, parturition or pharmacological stress from histamine, caffeine, beta-blockade or glucocorticoids. Attacks have a variable frequency, and the majority (80 per cent) last for less than an hour. Less commonly, patients with familial tumours are normotensive.

A direct relationship between high levels of catecholamines and myocardial injury exists with the potential for myocarditis and acute LVF.

Diagnosis is made simply through a 24-hour urine collection for urinary metanephrines. To improve the specificity of this test, patients should have monoamine oxidase inhibitors and mixed alpha- and beta-blockers (labetalol, carvedilol) discontinued beforehand. The tumour may be localized by CT scanning with the occasional need for radioisotope localization with MIBG. Where possible, phaeochromocytoma should be resected with careful pre- and peri-operative alpha-adrenoceptor blockade (with intravenous phentolamine at 5–10 µg/min) to diminish vasoconstriction and to allow intravascular volume expansion.

Hypertensive emergencies in pregnancy

The term gestational hypertension now covers the clinical syndrome of new-onset hypertension in the last trimester of pregnancy. The term eclampsia refers to the development of convulsions as a consequence of acute gestational hypertension (pre-eclampsia). Gestational hypertension is more common in primigravida and in situations where there are racial differences between parents. Predisposing variables include older maternal age, black race, multiple gestations, concomitant renal disease and pre-existing hypertension. It is a self-limiting condition with resolution after delivery and is characterized by sudden weight gain and oedema, retinal oedema, proteinuria and an increased plasma urate. An increased susceptibility to hypertensive encephalopathy exists due to the lack of previous hypertension in the mother and thus a breakthrough of increased cerebral blood flow from autoregulation which may lead to cerebral oedema and seizures.

The unifying cause of gestational hypertension is a reduction in utero-placental perfusion and subsequent decrease in prostaglandin production, and prostacyclin in particular. Although there was a vogue for the use of low-dose aspirin (<100 mg) to inhibit thromboxane production and prevent the development of gestational hypertension, this approach remains controversial given the increased risk of excessive bleeding during delivery.

The traditional approach to management has been bed rest and drug therapy with methyldopa, given its long-term safety profile in pregnancy, with the use of intravenous hydralazine around the time of delivery. However, beta-blockers, the alpha-blocker prazosin, labetalol and nifedipine have also been used with success. Furthermore, intravenous magnesium should be given in pre-eclampsia to prevent the development of seizure activity. A concern with the use of drugs, particularly beta-blockade, in mild gestational hypertension is the risk of intrauterine growth retardation with little effect on blood pressure control compared to simple bed rest alone. Should eclampsia supervene, patients should receive intravenous diazepam immediately to control seizure activity. Haemodynamic monitoring is recommended given the need to optimize intravascular volume status in the presence of oliguria (fluid challenge) or increased loading conditions (vasodilatation).

Hypertensive emergencies in critical illness

In critical illness, there are many factors which can increase catecholamine production and increase vasoconstriction leading to an acute elevation of blood pressure. Post-anaesthetic sympathomimetic stimulation, fluid overload and hypothermia are common causes of hypertension in critically ill patients. Hypertensive crises may occur in up to 5 per cent of intensive care unit patients. These may be treated by non-pharmacological means in the first instance over a period of 15 minutes, although these measures are likely to be effective only in a minority of patients. Such treatments include the relief of anxiety, pain or both; correction of hypoxia; patient instrumentation adjustment such as of mechanical ventilation and nasogastric tubes or urinary catheters; and correction of circulating blood volume and electrolyte imbalance. Where this proves to be ineffective, sublingual nifedipine 10 mg may be given as an initial treatment before intravenous therapy is considered.

KEY POINTS

- In about 1 per cent of patients with hypertension, an accelerated phase may occur as part of the progression of the disease and is commonest in the young black male population. It is commoner in secondary forms of the disease such as with phaeochromocytoma and in renovascular hypertension.

- Prior to established antihypertensive therapy, less than 25 per cent of patients with malignant hypertension survived 1 year, with a 1 per cent 5-year survival. In the current era with renal dialysis support, 1- and 5-year survival is 90 per cent and 80 per cent, respectively. Early death tends to occur due to stroke or acute renal failure.

- Malignant hypertension is the clinical syndrome where a sudden increased systemic blood pressure is likely to result in acute end-organ injury. The likelihood of this may vary according to pre-existing levels and to the rate of the acute rise, although it is accepted that a persistent diastolic blood pressure of greater than 130 mmHg is likely to result in vascular injury.

- The clinical features of a hypertensive crisis comprise a diastolic blood pressure greater than 130–140 mmHg, hypertensive retinopathy, hypertensive encephalopathy, acute renal failure and microangiopathic haemolytic anaemia (Table 4.2).

- Hypertensive encephalopathy is an acute medical emergency characterized by headache, irritability and an altered conscious level. Other potential complications of a hypertensive crisis are an intracerebral or subarachnoid haemorrhage and a thrombotic infarction in an individual with predisposing atherosclerotic cerebrovascular disease.

- Acute LVF is a common cardiovascular manifestation of a hypertensive crisis. Acute aortic dissection and acute coronary syndrome may also occur.

Table 4.2 Clinical manifestations of hypertensive crisis

- a diastolic blood pressure greater than 130 mmHg
- hypertensive retinopathy
  - haemorrhage, exudates and papilloedema (grades 3 and 4 hypertensive retinopathy)
- hypertensive encephalopathy
  - headache, confusion, altered consciousness, leading to seizure activity and coma
- acute renal failure
  - protein and red blood cells noted on urinalysis
  - hypokalaemia from secondary hyperaldosteronism
  - oliguria may ensue
- microangiopathic haemolytic anaemia

- A hypertensive emergency patient should be managed in a high-dependency environment with withdrawal of any potential treatments which may be exacerbating the situation. Treatment should be initiated by the intravenous route and titrated against antihypertensive response. Combination drug therapy is preferred to achieve an additive effect and may be tailored towards any compromise in a particular end-organ.

- Sodium nitroprusside (a short-acting arterial and venous dilator) is a first-line therapy for a hypertensive emergency. It has an immediate effect and its dose may be titrated against its efficacy and allow the administration of oral antihypertensive agents to allow discontinuation before the risk of thiocyanate toxicity.

- Labetalol (a mixed alpha- and beta-adrenergic blocker) is the other mainstay of therapy in a hypertensive emergency given as bolus and intravenous infusion.

- Gestational hypertension is the clinical syndrome of new-onset hypertension in the last trimester of pregnancy. It is more common in primigravida and in situations where there are racial differences between parents. Predisposing variables include older maternal age, black race, multiple gestations, concomitant renal disease and pre-existing hypertension. It is self-limiting with resolution after delivery and is characterized by sudden weight gain and oedema, retinal oedema and proteinuria.

KEY REFERENCES

Bennett NM, Shea S. Hypertensive emergency: case criteria, socio-demographic profile, and previous case of 100 cases. *Am J Public Health* 1988; **78**: 636–42.

Calhoun DA, Oparil S. Treatment of hypertensive crisis. *N Engl J Med* 1990; **323**: 1177–83.

Cumming AM, Davies DL. Intravenous labetalol in hypertensive emergency. *Lancet* 1979; **i**: 929–30.

Finnerty FA. Hypertensive encephalopathy. *Am J Med* 1972; **52**: 672–8.

Koch-Weser J. Hypertensive emergencies. *N Engl J Med* 1974; **290**: 211–14.

Lucas MJ, Levenko KJ, Cunningham FG. A comparison of magnesium sulphate with phenytoin for the prevention of eclampsia. *N Engl J Med* 1995; **333**: 201–5.

Manger WM. An overview of phaeochromocytoma: history, current concepts, vagaries, and diagnostic challenges. *Ann NY Acad Sci* 2006; **1073**: 1–20.

Montgomery HE, Kiernan LA, Whotworth CE, et al. Inhibition of tissue angiotensin converting enzyme activity prevents malignant hypertension in TGR(mREN2)27. *J Hypertens* 1998; **16**: 635–43.

Pancioli AM. Hypertension management in neurologic emergencies. *Ann Emerg Med* 2008; **51**(3 Suppl): S24–7.

Perez MI, Musini VM, Wright JM. Pharmacological interventions for hypertensive emergencies. Cochrane Database Syst Rev 2008; **1**: CD003653. DOI: 10.1002/14651858.CD003653.pub3.

Schiff E, Peleg E, Goldenberg M, et al. The use of aspirin to reduce pregnancy-induced hypertension and lower the ratio of thromboxane A2 to prostacyclin in relatively high-risk pregnancies. *N Engl J Med* 1989; **321**: 351–7.

Shusterman NH, Elliott WJ, White WB. Fenoldopam, but not nitroprusside improves renal function in severely hypertensive patients with impaired renal function. *Am J Med* 1993; **95**: 161–8.

Vaughan CJ, Delanty N. Hypertensive emergencies. *Lancet* 2000; **356**: 411–17.

Wilson DJ, Wallin JD, Vlachakis ND. Intravenous labetalol in the treatment of severe hypertension and hypertensive emergencies. *Am J Med* 1983; **75**(Suppl): 95–102.

ACUTE AORTIC SYNDROMES

BACKGROUND

Epidemiology

Dissection of the thoracic aorta is one of the most dramatic acute medical emergencies with serious adverse consequences if not diagnosed and treated promptly and appropriately. It has been estimated that there are around 3 cases per 100 000 population per year, most commonly occurring in men aged between 50 and 70 years, and more often in the black population. On average, left untreated, 50 per cent of patients die within 48 hours (estimated at a 1–2 per cent mortality per hour from presentation) with 70 per cent dead at 1 week and 90 per cent dead at 3 months. Frequency peaks in the morning, possibly related to the circadian variation in blood pressure.

The International Registry of Acute Aortic Dissection (IRAD), established in 1996, has reported trends in the management and outcome of the condition.

Definition and classification

Thoracic aortic dissection has been classified on anatomical grounds with regard to the origin and extent of the dissection and this has major implications in the treatment of the condition. The thoracic aorta is most likely to dissect at either the ascending aorta or in the descending aorta just below the left subclavian artery. The original classification by DeBakey described three different types:

- **type I** – dissection in the ascending thoracic aorta extending round the arch into the descending aorta and into the abdomen;

- **type II** – dissection in the ascending thoracic aorta only with no distal extension past the innominate artery;
- **type III** – dissection in the descending thoracic aorta distal to the left subclavian artery. Retrograde extension may occasionally occur back into the thoracic aortic arch and ascending aorta. In one follow-up study of aortic dissection, this subtype was subclassified into IIIa (limited to thoracic aorta) and IIIb (extension into the abdominal aorta).

The natural history of types I and II are similar and have led to the simpler Stanford classification of:

- **type A**, where dissection arises in the ascending aorta irrespective of its extension; and
- **type B**, equivalent to DeBakey type III, but excluding dissections with retrograde extension into the arch.

Rarely, a three-channelled dissection can occur where dissection occurs twice in the natural history of an individual patient (A + B or B + B, rarely A + A) in whom there is usually a high incidence of Marfan's syndrome.

A more recent classification, the Svensson classification, is based on the pathophysiological features of the aortic lesion rather than its location:

- **class 1:** classic aortic dissection with true and false lumen associated with an intimal tear;
- **class 2:** intramural haemorrhage or haematoma;
- **class 3:** ulceration of aortic plaque following plaque rupture;
- **class 4:** subtle or discrete aortic dissection with bulging of the aortic wall;
- **class 5:** iatrogenic or traumatic aortic dissection, illustrated by a catheter-induced separation of the intima.

Pathophysiology

Contemporary information relating to clinical factors underlying aortic dissection in a large group of subjects is available from the IRAD database. Acute aortic dissection is strongly associated with systemic hypertension (due to a sustained high intraluminal pressure) and with advancing age, but less so with atherosclerosis per se. Cystic medial degeneration in the aortic wall is an intrinsic feature of several connective tissue disorders which are associated with dissection such as Marfan's syndrome, Ehlers–Danlos syndrome and, occasionally, giant cell aortitis. These patients are at particular risk of dissection, often at a young age. There is an increased association with a bicuspid aortic valve and coarctation of the aorta, and thus with Turner's syndrome as well as Noonan's syndrome. Dissection can be seen in the last trimester of pregnancy and at the site of a previous surgical aortotomy. The presence of atherosclerosis per se does not predispose to thoracic aortic dissection but is associated with saccular aneurysmal dilatation. However, rupture of an intimal plaque in older patients remains a mechanism for dissection. In younger patients, cocaine use is an emerging risk factor.

Degeneration of the collagen and elastin matrix within the aortic medial layer is the chief predisposition in most cases of aortic dissection. The direct mechanism of dissection is unclear as the same pathological process may occur either through intimal rupture with secondary dissection into media or primary medial haemorrhage with local disruption of the intima.

The formation of a tear in the aortic intima allows penetration of blood into the diseased medial layer at arterial pressure, separating the laminar plane of the media and dissecting the aortic wall. This dissection process may extend a variable distance, usually in an antegrade direction, but sometimes retrogradely from the site of the tear. The blood-filled space between the dissected layers of the aortic wall becomes the false lumen. Shear forces may cause further tears in the intimal flap, producing exit sites or additional entry sites for blood flow in the false lumen. Eventually, distension of the false lumen at systemic arterial pressure may cause the intimal flap to bow into the true lumen, thereby narrowing its calibre and distorting its shape. The circulation of any major arterial vessel can be compromised by the dissection process, leading to ischaemia. The aortic valve may be disrupted, leading to aortic regurgitation. The dissecting process may rupture through the adventitia at any point, commonly into the pericardial space or left pleural cavity.

An intimal tear is not absolute in the pathology of the dissecting process as both penetrating atherosclerotic ulceration and intramural haematoma formation may occur without a discernible intimal disruption (see below). It is likely that these conditions may be precursors of classical dissection rather than separate entities, and all three conditions should be considered as belonging to a spectrum of acute aortic syndromes.

CLINICAL MANIFESTATIONS OF AORTIC DISSECTION

Aortic dissection can mimic several different intrathoracic pathologies in the evolution of the symptoms and signs. The common clinical features are:

- **Severe chest pain**: this is the commonest symptom of dissection. It is as severe at its outset as at any other time and is unremitting. It is often described as 'tearing' in nature. The pain tends to migrate as the dissecting haematoma extends. Anterior chest pain is common with proximal dissection whereas interscapular pain is common in descending aortic dissection and may be in both areas where a type I dissection has occurred. Pain may be noted in the neck and jaw where the ascending aorta or arch is involved.

- **Vasovagal symptoms**: acute diaphoresis with sweating, apprehension and syncope are common.

- **Altered blood pressure**: many patients are hypertensive at presentation. Conversely, hypotension may occur through cardiac tamponade (from rupture of the intrapericardial aortic root or from inflammation of the pericardium), aortic rupture, or dissection in the head and neck vessels, leading to a reduced perfusion pressure in the brachial artery (pseudohypotension) and thus pulse deficits. Pulse deficits are commonly associated with proximal dissection in the brachiocephalic vessels or less commonly through involvement of the left subclavian artery from a distal dissection. The loss of a pulse may occur either through an occlusive intimal flap at a vascular orifice or through direct compression of an artery lumen.

- **Aortic valve regurgitation**: this occurs either through a circumferential tear opening up the annulus and reducing coaptation, distortion of the valve apparatus through asymmetric dissection, or through direct disruption of the annular support, leading to a flail leaflet. It occurs in up to two-thirds of proximal dissection. If severe, acute left ventricular failure may ensue from acute aortic insufficiency.

- **Right coronary artery dissection**: leading to an acute inferior myocardial infarction (MI).

- **Acute neurological deficits**: ischaemic stroke, altered consciousness and paraparesis due to spinal cord ischaemia are most common with proximal dissections.

- **Mediastinal complications**: these occur through the expansion of the dissection with compression of the superior cervical sympathetic ganglion (Horner's syndrome), compression of the left recurrent laryngeal nerve (hoarseness), superior vena caval compression and tracheal compression.

- **Pleural effusion**: usually occurs on the left and is due to either rupture into the pleural space or an inflammatory exudate.

- **Acute rupture**: in addition to the pericardial space and pleural and intra-abdominal cavities, haemorrhage into the lung, oesophagus or rupture into right atrium may, rarely, occur.

- **Visceral infarction**: mesenteric and renal infarction may occur in dissections spreading into the abdominal aorta.

DIAGNOSIS OF AORTIC DISSECTION

Sudden onset of chest pain is common in several acute cardiovascular disorders. Because symptoms may mimic more common disorders such as ACS or acute pulmonary embolism (PE), and because characteristic physical findings such as a pulse deficit may be absent, dissection may be difficult to diagnose. It should be suspected in any patient presenting with chest or interscapular pain and diaphoresis.

Diagnosis is established with multi-slice computed tomography (MSCT), although transoesophageal echocardiogram (TOE) was the preferred diagnostic method in some places as it is portable, rapidly performed, sensitive and specific, and does not require the use of contrast agents. The choice of imaging modality should be determined by availability and expertise within individual centres. Where clinical suspicion is high, failure to diagnose dissection by one modality should prompt further investigation with another technique.

The important diagnostic investigational features are:

- **12-lead ECG**: this may be within normal limits or may show evidence of left ventricular hypertrophy due to commonly associated hypertension. If the dissection flap occludes one of the coronary ostia, this will produce ST elevation consitent with myocardial infarction. The right coronary ostium is more frequently invoved than the left.

- **Chest x-ray**: a widened mediastinum is a classical finding in thoracic aortic dissection. There may be an additional local bulge at the site of dissection. The presence of a left pleural effusion and tracheal deviation is often seen. Separation of calcification in the aortic arch from the apparent adventitial border is a powerful sign of dissection. However, extensive dissection can occur in the presence of a normal chest x-ray.

- **Echocardiography**: transthoracic echocardiography (TTE) may detect a proximal dissection where a dilated aortic root is present but is limited in any further delineation of a dissection. The accuracy of this assessment is also limited by the echogenicity of the patient. However, even if a flap is not identified, TTE can readily demonstrate several high-risk associated features of dissection: aortic root dilatation; presence and severity of aortic regurgitation (as well as revealing the presence of e.g. bicuspid valves); pericardial effusion; left ventricular regional wall motion abnormalities (implying coronary ostial occlusion). TOE allows visualization of the aortic root, proximal ascending aorta and descending aorta. With colour-flow Doppler, entry and exit sites between true and false lumen may be identified. With intramural haematoma, an echolucent crescentic region should be seen over a length of the aorta. Occasionally, the haematoma is circumferential and can be difficult to differentiate from common atherosclerotic thickening. A disadvantage is its limited ability to visualize the distal ascending aorta and proximal arch due to interposition of the trachea and left main bronchus. Furthermore, TOE is unable to image beyond the distal thoracic descending aorta and thus cannot assess the iliac vessels – an important limitation where endoluminal repair is being considered.

- **Multi-slice computed tomography**: MSCT with an intravenous contrast injection to enhance the intraluminal phase is the investigation of choice in most acute medical environments, given a reported sensitivity and specificity approaching 100 per cent. With the presence of a membrane (intimal flap), the false and true lumina can be identified. The false lumen is usually the larger of the two. Tomographic imaging enhances the diagnostic accuracy by demonstrating an abnormal tissue signature, although it is unable to provide haemodynamic information, and it relies upon the use of potentially nephrotoxic contrast agents, and may be unable to depict branch-vessel involvement. MSCT is also useful in the follow-up of dissection by allowing detailed assessment of early and late changes after surgery or medical treatment such as post-operative complications, healing of intramural haematoma, progression of intramural haematoma, and aneurysms of the true and false lumina. Monitoring of compromised abdominal branch vessels may be performed. CT angiography can demonstrate complex spatial relationships, mural abnormalities and extraluminal pathologies.

- **Magnetic resonance imaging**: MRI may be used as an alternative imaging technology without the need for contrast and with enhanced resolution. MRI gives an improved anatomic delineation of the aorta and can provide high-quality images in several planes, including a left anterior oblique view that displays the entire thoracic aorta. Furthermore, MRI is superior to conventional CT in differentiating acute intramural haematoma from atherosclerotic plaque and chronic intraluminal thrombus, which is important where there is diagnostic uncertainty.

- **Aortic angiography:** with the improvements made in echocardiographic and tomographic imaging, invasive confirmation of dissection is no longer performed. The intention of angiography was to identify the site of origin and to delineate the extent of the dissection. The procedure carried with it a significant mortality, and currently should only be performed for cases where the diagnosis is uncertain after other imaging. It is of no help in the diagnosis of intramural haematoma.

There is increasing interest in the identification of highly sensitive and specific biomarkers that may aid diagnosis of aortic dissection. Markers under scrutiny include D-dimers, elastin fragments and smooth-muscle myosin heavy-chain protein. D-dimer assay, widely used in the diagnosis of acute PE, seems to be potentially useful as a rule-out test in aortic dissection.

TREATMENT OF AORTIC DISSECTION

It is the course and propogation of the dissection rather than the intimal tear itself that leads to the complications of acute aortic dissection. For this reason, the modern surgical management of a proximal dissection has focused on excising the intimal tear and obliterating the false lumen by oversewing the aortic edges, thus removing the driving force behind the propagation of the false channel. An interposition graft may be required in the ascending aorta to restore integrity to this section of the dissection. If the aortic valve is competent and unaffected directly by the dissection, it may be resuspended in the graft at the aortic valve ring or it may require replacement with a prosthesis if disrupted. Simultaneously, systemic blood pressure and left ventricular contractility should be significantly reduced to remove the direct pulsatile stress on the aortic wall.

Immediate therapy

All patients in whom a thoracic aortic dissection is suspected should be monitored and treated in a high-dependency environment for haemodynamic and cardiac rhythm monitoring and for central venous access. Patients should be cross-matched for the eventuality of either dissection or rupture and early surgery. The three initial goals of therapy are:

(1) to alleviate pain with intravenous opiate analgesia.

(2) to reduce systolic pressure to a range of 100–120 mmHg, equivalent to a mean arterial pressure of 60–75 mmHg, and sufficient to maintain vital organ perfusion.

(3) to reduce the velocity of left ventricular ejection (the dP/dt) by beta-blockade independently of systemic blood pressure lowering.

Blood pressure lowering is achieved by an infusion of intravenous sodium nitroprusside up to a maximum dose of 400 μg/min (5 μg/kg/min). The infusion should not be given for more than 48 hours due to the risk of cyanide toxicity. Frequent blood gases should be taken for acid–base status (a metabolic acidosis tends to develop with cyanide toxicity). Concomitant infusion of vitamin B_{12} (hydroxocobalamin) reduces plasma cyanide levels through the formation of cyanocobalamin. Sodium nitroprusside reduces the blood pressure but may actually increase the dP/dt through afterload reduction. Intravenous beta-blockade is used to reduce dP/dt. The most popular agent used is labetalol, which is a non-selective beta-blocker and alpha-blocker. It can be given either as bolus doses of 5–20 mg up to a total of 300 mg or may be given as an infusion (see Appendix A). Beta-blockers (and other rate-limiting agents) should be used with caution if severe aortic regurgitation is present.

Definitive treatment

The accepted paradigm in dissection management is that surgical treatment is superior to medical treatment in the management of type A dissection, whereas medical therapy is superior in uncomplicated type B dissection (see Box 5.1). This comes about through surgery preventing progression of dissection and potentially fatal consequences. Patients with distal dissection tend to be older with atherosclerotic vascular disease, often with a reduced cardiac reserve, and tend to tolerate surgery less well, favouring medical therapy. The attrition rate in patients with proximal dissection treated surgically occurs through complications having already occurred or through the friability of the aortic wall at surgery.

In practice, the decision to intervene in chronic dissection is based upon evidence of progressive pathological change over time. In patients with symptoms or signs of peripheral ischaemia, the indication for intervention is clear. In asymptomatic individuals, intervention is recommended for progressive aortic dilatation (>5 cm maximum diameter), and when there is evidence of a persistent false lumen in communication with the true lumen.

Box 5.1 Indications for specific treatment of aortic dissection

Surgery
- Acute type A dissection
- Acute type B dissection with complications
  - compromised perfusion to vital organs
  - rupture/ threatened rupture
  - retrograde dissection to ascending aorta/aortic valve regurgitation
  - Marfan's syndrome
  - inability or control pain
  - saccular aneurysm formation
- Chronic dissection with complications
  - progressive aortic dilatation (>50 mm maximum diameter)
  - persistent false lumen in communication with the true lumen
  - persistent pain

Medical therapy
- Uncomplicated type B dissection
- Uncomplicated arch dissection
- Stable chronic dissection

Surgery

Current practice dictates that the proximal dissection should be repaired early to prevent extension and rupture, and to operate on distal dissections extending proximally using cardiopulmonary bypass. Of patients with type A dissections, the IRAD database revealed lower 30-day mortality in surgically treated patients than those treated medically (see Clinical outcomes in aortic dissection).

The goal of surgery is to prevent progression of the dissection and to relieve obstruction in peripheral branches: thus, the intimal tear is excised and the origin of the false lumen excluded by proximal and distal suturing of the edges of the aorta. A prosthetic Dacron graft may be needed to approximate the ends of the aorta. Surgery requires a period of deep hypothermic circulatory arrest. Where the aortic valve is involved, the false channel is decompressed by the surgery described above, but may still require replacement or repair. Where the aorta is very friable, the whole ascending aorta and valve may be replaced using a composite graft containing a prosthesis with resuturing of the coronary arteries to the conduit. Preservation of the native aortic valve, which avoids the complications associated with a prosthetic valve, usually requires approximation of the two layers of dissected aortic wall and resuspension of the commissures with pledgeted sutures. However, prosthetic valve replacement is frequently advisable in the setting of pre-existent valve disease or in Marfan's syndrome to reduce the likelihood of re-operation.

Surgical fenestration has been used as a means of decompressing an occlusive false lumen in the descending aorta in patients with visceral or limb ischaemia. Fenestration may be performed alongside ascending aortic surgery and additional abdominal aortic grafting. It should ideally be performed within 48 hours of presentation to prevent thrombotic occlusion of the false lumen. In one series, surgical fenestration in decending aortic dissection was associated with mortality rates of 77 and 53 per cent at 3 and 5 years, respectively. Fenestration can also be done percutaneously and is usually done in the pararenal or infrarenal area (see below).

Percutaneous interventional treatment

In type B dissection, the persistence of a false lumen has an adverse effect of clinical outcome (higher rates of re-operation and mortality) where an active communication persists between true and false lumina, compared to where there is thrombosis of the false lumen. The deployment of balloon-expandable or self-expanding endoluminal stents may be performed to re-establish flow into branch vessels compromised by dissection into the origin of the vessel. If a branch vessel is compromised by pressure from the false lumen over the origin of the vessel, a fenestration procedure may be undertaken to decompress the false lumen. Similarly, endoluminal exclusion with a stent graft prosthesis (consisting of circumferential nitinol stent springs arranged as a tube and covered with a Dacron or polytetrafluoroethylene [PTFE] graft exterior) placed over the false lumen entry site will decompress the false lumen, causing the flap to oppose the aortic wall and relieve branch vessel compromise. The advantage of endoluminal exclusion in acute dissection is that it combines closure of the false lumen and prevents subsequent dilatation with relief of branch vessel obstruction.

Stent grafts are sized by measurement from pre-procedure imaging. They require a proximal neck of ideally 20 mm of 'normal aorta' above the false lumen origin to ensure secure deployment against the aortic wall. The potential for ischaemia through occlusion of the left subclavian artery may be predicted by preliminary occlusive balloon inflation for 20 minutes at its origin to assess the integrity of the collateral circulation, perhaps using a partially covered graft if necessary. The position of the undeployed graft may be obtained using aortography, intravascular ultrasound or TOE. The distal neck may be normal supracoeliac aorta or biluminal descending thoracic aorta. In the absence of a distal neck, the shortest graft that effectively covers the entry site is used.

These techniques are being increasingly used in type B dissections, particularly when complications ensue. Short-term results from stenting may appear encouraging, with overall major events seen in 11 per cent, including in-hospital mortality of 5 per cent, stroke rate of 2 per cent, paraplegia in 1 per cent. Further, 2 per cent of cases were complicated by transformation to type A dissection. The INvestigation of STEnt grafts in patients with type B Aortic Dissection (INSTEAD) trial compared the use of covered stents with medical therapy alone for uncomplicated type B dissection. Short-term results at 12 months indicated equivalent mortality in patients with uncomplicated acute type B dissection who were treated with conventional medical therapy alone or with endovascular stenting. Registry data relating to 180 patients treated with the endovascular Talent thoracic stent graft for acute or chronic aortic dissection are also available. Intermediate term (mean 22 months) follow-up yielded survival rates of 91 per cent and 82 per cent at 24 and 36 months, respectively. Emergency status (vs elective cases) was an independent predictor of major adverse events. Analysis of the IRAD database suggests that endovascular treatment seems to provide better in-hospital survival in patients with acute type B dissection: in-hospital complications occurred in 20 per cent of patients treated with an endovascular technique and in 40 per cent of patients who underwent open surgical repair. In-hospital mortality was significantly higher after open surgery than after endovascular treatment with a three-fold increase in risk for open surgical repair.

Thus, there are many uncertainties relating to use of stent-graft techniques in aortic dissection. A key question to be answered by furture studies is whether there is any role for stenting with or without conventional surgery for type A dissections.

As described above, the fenestration technique may be employed using an endovascular approach (usually as a bridge to definitive endoluminal repair) using a needle to pass a guide wire through the intimal flap, then balloon dilatation of the puncture site. Several fenestrations can be performed in order to equalize pressures in the true and false lumina, and stenting of branches may be performed to optimize flow. In cases where endoluminal repair or fenestration is considered, digital subtraction angiography, or magnetic resonance angiography, is an essential prelude to allow assessment of the access arteries (usually the iliacs), measurement of the aorta to permit selection of the correct device length and diameter, confirmation of branch vessel involvement and biluminal manometry prior to fenestration.

PENETRATING ATHEROSCLEROTIC ULCERATION AND INTRAMURAL AORTIC HAEMATOMA

These entities are radiologically distinct from classical dissection, with no intimal flap evident. In penetrating atherosclerotic ulcers (PAU), a visible crater extends into the aortic wall and is associated with haematoma within the media of the aortic wall. An intramural haematoma (IMH) is present where significant thickening or enhancement of the aortic wall is seen in the absence of a flap or dissection. The clinical features of these two variants may differ from dissection. Patients with PAU/IMH are older than patients with both type A and B dissections, and thus are commonest between the seventh and ninth decades. Patients with PAU/IMH are almost always hypertensive (94 per cent). PAU and IMH are most common in the descending aorta (90 per cent and 71 per cent, respectively). PAU and IMH tend to occur in more dilated aortas and have an association with abdominal aortic aneurysms. The presentation with anterior or posterior chest pain is similar to, and may be indistinguishable from, that of classical dissection. In one review of over 200 cases presenting as aortic dissection, one-eighth of cases were reclassified to either PAU or IMH. However, PAU/IMH generally do not cause arterial vessel compromise and thus distal limb ischaemia or visceral compromise, and tend to be focal without propagation.

Penetrating atherosclerotic ulceration

Penetrating ulcers occur within severely atherosclerotic, frequently calcified descending thoracic or abdominal aortae, in contrast to classical dissection, which is more often associated with hypertension. Ulcers are generally focal lesions appearing as an irregular outpouching of the aortic wall. Ulceration may precede both IMH or dissection; dissection following PAU is usually shorter, and contained by neighbouring fibrosis and calcification, with a thicker flap. When compared to dissection and IMH, PAU is most commonly associated with aortic rupture. Optimal treatment of PAU is yet to be established. Medical treatment has been shown to be effective in most patients; additionally, several registries have shown favourable outcomes with open surgery and endovascular repair in selected patients. A large series of patients presenting with PAU identified rupture at presentation as the main indicator of medical failure. Therefore these patients are more likely to benefit from early intervention. Patients who are asymptomatic or found to have PAU as an incidental finding rarely require intervention but should be followed up for any progressive increase in size of the ulcer.

Intramural aortic haematoma

IMH occurs when blood accumulates in the vessel media in the absence of a flap. Formation of an IMH may follow rupture of the vasa vasorum, or from extension of a PAU (which is identified in 20 per cent of IMH). Extension of IMH towards the intima may lead to a tear and subsequent dissection. It is thought likely that the radial level in the wall at which an IMH occurs determines whether an acute dissection or haematoma develops. It may be that if blood collects closer to the adventitia, there is less likelihood of intimal rupture. This would also explain a higher external rupture rate with IMH, which tends to run a more malignant course than typical descending aortic dissection.

The diagnosis of IMH requires identification of an expanded aortic wall, usually <15 mm, without a connection with the aortic lumen. Echocardiographically, an aortic wall thickness of >7 mm is diagnostic; there may be echo-lucent zones seen within a crescentic aortic wall thickening.

The classification of IMH is similar to that of classical aortic dissection (Stanford A and B according to involvement of the ascending aorta), and this influences management as with true dissection. A meta-analysis of 168 patients with IMH has shown that around one-quarter of type A IMH progressed to dissection or rupture. Overall, the 30-day mortality with surgery was 18 per cent compared to 60 per cent with medical treatment. In contrast, medical treatment improved mortality compared to surgery in type B patients (8 per cent vs 33 per cent, respectively). Accordingly, type B IMH may be successfully managed by medical treatment alone, with beta-blockers the mainstay of treatment where possible. However, there are certain features which portend an adverse prognosis in IMH even without ascending aorta or arch involvement (Box 5.2) Unfortunately, surgical intervention for type B IMH may be complicated by paraplegia owing to disruption of blood flow to the spinal arteries. Endovascular stenting in this setting is an emerging option, particularly for localized lesions associated with PAU, although the precise role is currently unclear.

Box 5.2 High-risk features in aortic intramural haematoma

- Type A intramural haematoma
- Increased aortic diameter (>50 mm)
- Haematoma thickness >11 mm
- Recurrent chest pain
- Progressive enlargement
- Penetrating finger-like projections
- Pleural or pericardial fluid
- Associated ulcer with diameter >20 mm or depth >10 mm

Adapted with permission from Bolger AF *Heart* 2008; **94**: 1670–4.

CLINICAL OUTCOME IN AORTIC DISSECTION

From the International Registry of Acute Aortic Dissection, overall in-hospital mortality was 27.4 per cent:

- **Type A**
  - surgical management 26 per cent
  - medical management 58 per cent

- **Type B**
  - surgical management 31 per cent
  - medical management 11 per cent

These high mortality rates have been confirmed in several other large series. Moreover, for acute disease complicated by end-organ ischaemia, surgical mortality exceeds 50 per cent, with a substantial risk (7–36 per cent) of paraplegia (or paresis), dependent upon the extent of aortic dissection and the duration of cross-clamping, amongst those who survive. Chronic aortic dissection (presentation up to 2 weeks after the onset of symptoms) has a higher in-hospital survival of around 90 per cent whether they are treated medically or surgically, largely through self-selection due to the lack of acute complications in the initial phase of dissection.

The initial success of surgical or medical therapy is usually sustained at long-term follow-up with typical 5-year survival rates of 75–82 per cent. A number of clinical factors have been linked with poor prognosis in addition to the anatomy of the dissection. Acute complications at the time of acute presentation, such as a cerebrovascular accident, MI, severe aortic regurgitation, renal failure, mesenteric infarction and lower limb ischaemia, in addition to aneurysmal dilatation of the dissected aorta and increasing age, predict an adverse outcome.

The incidence of aneurysm formation at a site remote from the original surgical repair is 17–25 per cent, with the majority appearing within 2 years. Many arise from dilatation of the residual false lumen in the distal unresected aortic segments and are prone to rupture owing to their relatively thin outer wall. To identify such a development, careful long-term follow-up with serial aortic imaging, usually using MRI, is recommended. Patients are at highest risk during the first 2 years and should be assessed every 3–6 months during this period. Thereafter, they should be re-evaluated every 6–12 months according to their perceived individual risk.

KEY POINTS

- Acute aortic dissection in a high-mortality condition with a 48-hour mortality of 50 per cent, with 70 per cent dead at 1 week and 90 per cent dead at 3 months, if left untreated. With treatment, overall hospital mortality is 27 per cent.

- Acute thoracic dissection is strongly associated with systemic hypertension and with advancing age. Several connective tissue disorders (of which Marfan's syndrome is the commonest) are associated with dissection due to cystic medial degeneration in the aortic wall.

- There are pathological variations accounting for one-eighth of cases of 'aortic dissection'. In penetrating atherosclerotic ulcers (PAU), no intimal flap is demonstrable with a crater visible extending into the aortic wall associated with haematoma within the media of the aortic wall. IMH occurs where significant thickening or enhancement of the aortic wall is seen in the absence of a flap or dissection.

- Aortic dissection can mimic different conditions in the evolution of the symptoms and signs such as severe chest pain, vasovagal symptoms and hypotension, severe hypertension, acute aortic regurgitation, myocardial infarction, stroke, pleural effusion and visceral infarction.

- The diagnosis is most accurately done with spiral computed tomography (with contrast enhancement), although TOE has been an alternative in many centres as it is portable, rapidly performed, sensitive and specific, and does not require the use of contrast agents. MRI gives an improved anatomic delineation of the aorta and can provide high-quality images in several planes. Prior to definitive imaging, high-risk features can be picked up with transthoracic echocardiography.

- Patients in whom thoracic aortic dissection is suspected should be monitored and treated in a high-dependency environment, and prepared for the possibility of early surgery. The two initial goals of therapy are pain relief and the reduction of the systolic pressure to a range of 100–120 mmHg (equivalent to a mean arterial pressure of 60–75 mmHg and sufficient to maintain vital organ perfusion). Where possible, left ventricular contractility should be reduced by beta-blockade independently of systemic blood pressure lowering.

- Urgent surgery is indicated in ascending thoracic aortic dissection and in descending thoracic aortic dissection where there are complications such as visceral ischaemia, threatened rupture and retrograde dissection to ascending aorta.

KEY REFERENCES

Ahmad F, Cheshire N, Hamady M. Acute aortic syndromes: pathology and therapeutic strategies. *Postgrad Med. J* 2006; **82**: 305–12.

Anangostopoulos CE, Prabhakar MJS, Kittle CF. Aortic dissections and dissecting aneurysms. *Am J Cardiol* 1972; **30**: 263–73.

Bolger AF. Aortic intramural haematoma. *Heart* 2008; **94**: 1670–4.

Cambria RP, Brewster DC, Gertler J, et al. Vascular complications associated with spontaneous aortic dissection. *J Vasc Surg* 1988; **7**: 199–209.

Casselaman FP, Tan ES, Vermeulen FE, et al. Durability of aortic valve preservation and root reconstruction in acute type A aortic dissection. *Ann Thorac Surg* 2000; **70**: 1227–33.

Coady MA, Rizzo JA, Elefteriades JA. Pathologic variants of thoracic aortic dissections: penetrating atherosclerotic ulcers and intramural hematomas. *Cardiol Clin* 1999; **17**: 637–57.

Daily PO, Trueblood HW, Stinson EB, Wuerflein RD, Shumway NE. Management of acute aortic dissection. *Ann Thorac Surg* 1970; **10**: 237–47.

Dake MD, Kato N, Mitchell S, et al. Endovascular stent-graft placement for the treatment of acute aortic dissection. *N Engl J Med* 1999; **340**: 1546–52.

DeBakey ME, McCollum CH, Crawford ES, et al. Dissection and dissecting aneurysms of the aorta: 20-year follow-up of 527 patients treated surgically. *Surgery* 1982; **92**: 1118–34.

Doroghazi RM, Slater EE, DeSanctis RW, et al. Long-term survival of patients with treated aortic dissection. *J Am Coll Cardiol* 1984; **3**: 1026–34.

Erbel R, Oelert H, Meyer J, et al. Effect of medical and surgical therapy on aortic dissection evaluated by transoesophageal echocardiography. Implications for prognosis and therapy. *Circulation* 1993; **87**: 1604–15.

Ergin MA, Phillips RA, Galla JD, et al. Significance of distal false lumen after type A dissection repair. *Ann Thorac Surg* 1994; **57**: 820–5.

Fattori R, Tsai TT, Myrmel T, et al. Complicated acute type B dissection: is surgery still the best option?: a report from the International Registry of Acute Aortic Dissection. *JACC Cardiovasc Interv* 2008; **1**: 395–402.

Golledge J, Eagle KA. Acute aortic dissection. *Lancet* 2008; **372**: 55–66.

Hagan PG, Nienaber CA, Isselbacher EM, et al. The International Registry of Acute Aortic Dissection (IRAD). New insights into an old disease. *JAMA* 2000; **283**: 897–903.

Heinemann M, Laas J, Karck M, Borst HG. Thoracic aortic aneurysms after type A aortic dissection: necessity for follow-up. *Ann Thorac Surg* 1990; **49**: 580–4.

Kaji S, Nishigami K, Akasada T, et al. Prediction of progression or regression of type A aortic intramural hematoma by computed tomography. *Circulation* 1999; **100**(Suppl 19): II281–6.

Khandheria BK. Aortic dissection. The last frontier. *Circulation* 1993; **87**: 1765–7.

Kieffer E, Koskas F, Godet G, et al. Treatment of aortic arch dissection using the elephant trunk technique. *Ann Vasc Surg* 2000; **14**: 612–19.

Kolff J, Bates RJ, Balderman SC, Shenkoya K, Anagnostopoulos CE. Acute aortic arch dissection: re-evaluation of the indication for medical and surgical therapy. *Am J Cardiol* 1977; **39**: 727–33.

Masuda Y, Yamada Z, Morooka N, Watanabe S, Inagaki Y. Prognosis of patients with medically treated dissections. *Circulation* 1991; **84**: III7–13.

Meredith EL, Masani ND. Echocardiography in the emergency assessment of acute aortic syndromes. *Eur J Echocardiogr* 2009; **10**: i31–9.

Miller DC. The continuing dilemma concerning medical versus surgical management of patients with acute type B dissections. *Semin Thorac Cardiovasc Surg* 1993; **5**: 33–46.

Miller DC, Stinson EB, Oyer PE, et al. Operative treatment of aortic dissections. Experience with 125 patients over a sixteen-year period. *J Thorac Cardiovasc Surg* 1979; **78**: 365–81.

Moriyama Y, Yotsumoto G, Kuriwaki K, et al. Intramural haematoma of the thoracic aorta. *Eur J Cardiothorac Surg* 1998; **13**: 230–9.

Nienaber CA, von Kodolitsch Y, Petersen B, et al. Intramural haemorrhage of the thoracic aorta: diagnostic and therapeutic implications. *Circulation* 1995; **92**: 1465–72.

Nienaber CA, Fattori R, Lund G, et al. Nonsurgical reconstruction of thoracic aortic dissection by stent-graft placement. *N Engl J Med* 1999; **340**: 1539–45.

Paneton JM, The SH, Cherry KJ, et al. Aortic fenestration for acute or chronic aortic dissection. *J Vasc Surg* 2000; **32**: 711–21.

Pate JW, Richardson RJ, Eastridge CE. Acute aortic dissection. *Ann Surg* 1976; **42**: 395–404.

Pradhan S, Elefteriades JA, Sumpio BE. Utility of the aortic fenestration technique in the management of acute aortic dissections. *Ann Thorac Cardiovasc Surg* 2007; **13**: 296–300.

Rapezi C, Rocchi G, Fattori R, et al. Usefulness of transoesophageal echocardiographic monitoring to improve the outcome of stent-graft treatment of thoracic aortic aneurysms. *Am J Cardiol* 2001; **87**: 315–19.

Slonim SM, Miller DC, Mitchell RS, et al. Percutaneous balloon fenestration and stenting for life-threatening ischemic complications in patients with acute aortic dissection. *J Thorac Cardiovasc Surg* 1999; **117**: 1118–27.

Svensson LG, Labib SB, Eisenhau JR. Intimal tear without haematoma. *Circulation* 1999; **99**: 1331–6.

Vilacosta I, San Roman JA, Ferreiros J, et al. Natural history and serial morphology of aortic intramural haematoma: a novel variant of aortic dissection. *Am Heart J* 1997; **13**: 495–507.

von Kodolitsch Y, Csösz SK, Koschyk DH, et al. Intramural hematoma of the aorta: predictors of progression to dissection and rupture. *Circulation* 2003; **107**: 1158–63.

Yamada T, Tada S, Harada J. Aortic dissection without intimal rupture: diagnosis with MR imaging and CT. *Radiology* 1988; **168**: 347–52.

Yucel EK, Steinberg FL, Egglin TK, Geller SC, Waltman AC, Athanasoulis CA. Penetrating aortic ulcers: diagnosis with MR imaging. *Radiology* 1990; **177**: 779–81.

ACUTE PULMONARY EMBOLISM

BACKGROUND

Epidemiology

Venous thromboembolism (encompassing deep venous thrombosis [DVT] and pulmonary embolism [PE]) is a great constant in acute medicine with no major difference in its incidence or mortality in the past 20 years. The age- and sex-adjusted incidence rate is 117 cases per 100 000 person-years. The incidence rises particularly in those aged >60 years, irrespective of gender, largely driven by PE.

Pulmonary embolism is a life-threatening condition associated with a high mortality rate. There is a direct relationship between age and mortality. In almost a quarter of patients with PE, the initial clinical manifestation is sudden death. Mortality is at least 10 per cent in the first few hours of presentation and exceeds 15 per cent at 3 months post diagnosis. Unfortunately, PE is undiagnosed in many cases, and the majority of patients with fatal PE do not have specific symptoms to aid diagnosis. Indeed, PE occurs more frequently among patients with alternative causes of dyspnoea, such as those with heart failure and chronic obstructive airways disease. For example, the relative risk of PE in heart failure patients is twice that of those without heart failure, and increases as left ventricular systolic function declines. Furthermore, PE patients with heart failure have higher overall mortality and readmission rates than those without heart failure.

Pathophysiology of venous thromboembolism

Pulmonary emboli occur following dislodgment of a venous thrombus from the deep veins of the leg or the pelvic veins which travels into the pulmonary arterial circulation. The risk of PE with a proximal DVT above the calf is as high as 50 per cent, with a lower risk in thromboses confined to the calf.

The clinical signs of embolism are determined by:

(1) the level at which the thrombus is occlusive, and

(2) to what extent pulmonary blood flow is diminished.

Additional determinants of the clinical effect of embolism include the patient's pre-existing cardiorespiratory reserve, and the humoral effect of vasoactive factors such as serotonin and thromboxane A_2 released by activated platelets at the site of pulmonary artery occlusion. These peptides have a direct bronchoconstrictor effect in addition to a vasoconstrictor action, and can potentiate the increase in pulmonary hypertension due to mechanical effects of the thrombus.

The development of a venous thrombus is triggered by Virchow's triad of local injury, hypercoagulability and stasis of flow. A hypercoagulable state is commonly acquired, although there are a few rare primary conditions that predispose to a venous thrombus, usually in a younger age group (<45 years old) with an unexpected thromboembolism. Such hypercoagulable conditions exist in antithrombin III deficiency, protein C deficiency, protein S deficiency and in inherited conditions with defective tPA (tissue plasminogen activator) release. The presence of the 'lupus anticoagulant' (with or without systemic lupus) that interferes with phospholipid-dependent coagulation is associated with venous thrombosis. Some of these patients have anticardiolipin antibodies that paradoxically prolong the activated partial thromboplastin time (aPTT).

It is much commoner to see venous thromboembolism in certain clinical situations occurring secondary to acquired pro-thrombotic abnormalities in coagulation, in platelets and in venous blood flow. The commonest situations increasing risk for developing PE include:

- recent surgery, particularly orthopaedic procedures
- cancer, with venous thrombosis often occurring before overt malignancy
- an altered hormonal state, such as the early post-partum period in pre-eclampsia as well as the rare association with the oral contraceptive pill.

Table 6.1 Incidence of pulmonary embolism in different clinical situations

Clinical situation	Low risk	Intermediate risk	High risk
General surgery	Age <40 years Surgery <30 min No risk factors	Age 40–60 years Surgery 30–60 min	Age >60 years Surgery >60 min + risk factors
Orthopaedic surgery	Minor trauma	Leg plaster cast	Hip/knee surgery Hip fracture Multiple trauma
Medical conditions	Pregnancy	Heart failure Stroke Malignancy	Prolonged immobility
Incidence (%) Distal DVT Proximal DVT Symptomatic PE Fatal PE	 2% 0.4% 0.2% 0.002%	 10–40% 6–8% 1–2% 0.1–0.8%	 40–80% 10–15% 5–10% 1–5%

Adapted from Riedel (1996)

Platelet aggregation may be enhanced in heparin-induced thrombocytopenia and in myeolproliferative disorders leading to thrombosis. Similarly, patients with hyperviscosity syndromes (polycythaemia, leukaemia and sickle cell disease) are more likely to have thrombotic complications. Venous thrombosis is common in the nephrotic syndrome.

Venous stasis may also be promoted by mechanical variables such as immobilization with chronic illness and obesity. Prolonged central venous cannulation for long-term drug therapy or parenteral nutrition can lead to right atrial thrombus formation and subsequent embolism. The relative risk of pulmonary embolism in different clinical situations is shown in Table 6.1.

DIAGNOSIS OF DEEP VENOUS THROMBOSIS

Venous thromboembolism is a clinical situation where the diagnosis is more often not made than made. The clinical suspicion of a DVT (leg swelling, calf tenderness, venous distension of subcutaneous vessels, discolouration) should be confirmed objectively. This is necessary due to the lack of predictive accuracy in the clinical examination: calf pain has

66–91% sensitivity and 3–87% specificity for DVT. No single investigation for the diagnosis of DVT has ideal properties (100% sensitivity and specificity, low cost, no risk), and often several tests are performed, either sequentially or in combination. Contrast venography and pulmonary angiography for PE were the gold standards for diagnosis through default and are largely used for comparison in trials.

Investigations are often integrated with clinical criteria in order to construct diagnostic algorithms.

D-dimers. Plasma D-dimers are specific cross-linked fibrin derivatives, formed and released during fibrin degradation by plasmin; thus, concentrations are elevated with venous thromboembolism. Whilst sensitive for diagnosisng venous thromboembolism, elevated D-dimer levels are non-specific as they occur in other disorders (e.g. during infection, in malignancy, after surgery, in heart failure and in pregnancy). Nevertheless, D-dimer testing generally has a high negative predictive value, and is useful in excluding venous thromboembolism when combined with clinical probability assessment.

Compression ultrasound with venous imaging. In the current era, ultrasonography is the imaging test of choice in confirming suspected DVT. The combination of colour Doppler measurement of venous flow with 2D cross-sectional assessment of lower extremity veins is termed duplex ultrasound. It is non-invasive and portable, and can also identify other causes of calf/thigh symptoms (e.g. Baker's cysts, haematomas, lymphadenopathy, femoral artery aneurysm, superficial thrombophlebitis and abscesses). Compression of opposing venous walls is applied by the transducer, with the primary diagnostic criterion being the non-compressibility of a vein. The presence of intraluminal echogenic thrombus, venous distension, absence of a colour-flow Doppler signal and loss of phasic flow are secondary criteria. Its diagnostic accuracy is limited in pelvic and calf DVT, in recurrent DVT and in asymptomatic proximal DVT, as well as in the presence of severe obesity or oedema. Acute DVT may be differentiated from chronic DVT by an increased compressibility and reduced echogenicity of thrombus seen. Of note, however, ultrasound findings may not return to normal after a DVT, and ultrasonography may be less useful for diagnosing recurrent DVT. For proximal DVT, a sensitivity of 89–100% and specificity of 95–100% is reported with ultrasound. In the smaller, more anatomically variable calf veins, ultrasonographic sensitivity falls to 73–87%, with a specificity of 83–100%, dropping to a sensitivity of 33–58% in asymptomatic calf DVT.

Impedance plethysmography (IPG). This is a safe, non-invasive, operator-dependent, portable technique which may be used to screen for the presence of DVT, particularly in the proximal (rather than calf) deep veins. The test is based on the principle that the volume of blood in the leg affects its ability to conduct an applied current (inversely proportional to the impedance in two limb electrodes). Venous outflow is obstructed by a thigh cuff that causes a fall-off in impedance. Release of the cuff leads to an increase in proximal blood flow as well as impedance. If a DVT is present in a major vein from the popliteals to the iliacs, the rate of venous emptying (and increase in impedance) is slower. Studies have demonstrated sensitivities of 92–98% for symptomatic proximal DVT, compared to a sensitivity of only 20% for calf DVT. Negative IPG has been associated with a small rate of subsequent pulmonary embolism of around 2.5%. Thus, plethysmography is only useful for early recurrences where IPG normalization has been demonstrated.

Contrast venography. In light of improvements in ultrasound resolution, the need for invasive venography has diminished. It should be reserved for situations where the ultrasound examination is equivocal or normal despite a high clinical suspicion. With large extensive deep thromboses, the contrast injected in the foot may not reach the deep veins leading to a false-negative venogram. Disadvantages include its invasiveness, allergic reaction to dye, toxicity from contrast, and the test may rarely actually cause DVT through phlebitis. It is relatively contraindicated in acute renal failure and in critical peripheral vascular disease.

Magnetic resonance imaging (MRI). This has a high sensitivity for thrombus (up to 100%) and allows assessment of the pelvic veins and IVC in addition to the proximal veins in the thigh. Compared to contrast venography, it is less sensitive for calf DVT. It is non-invasive and not operator-dependent (but is reader-dependent) and allows assessment of extraneous pathologies. It is more expensive than other technologies and is precluded by metallic objects and morbid obesity/claustrophobia. Like venography, it should be undertaken if ultrasonography is either non-diagnostic or negative in the context of high clinical suspicion.

DIAGNOSIS OF ACUTE PULMONARY EMBOLISM

Clinical features

In patients with acute PE, unexplained dyspnoea (the most common presenting symptom), pleuritic chest pain and haemoptysis are classical symptoms. On examination, tachypnoea and tachycardia are common signs; other signs may include raised venous pressures, tricuspid regurgitation and a louder pulmonary second heart sound. Similarly, syncope or sudden hypotension may indicate a large clot burden.

However, the need for objective testing is necessary in the diagnosis of PE as the history and examination of the patient are non-specific. A systematic review of 18 diagnostic studies (comprising almost 6000 patients) assessed the value of various clinical features in diagnosing PE. The most useful features for ruling in PE were syncope, shock, thrombophlebitis, current DVT, leg swelling, sudden dyspnoea, active cancer, recent surgery, haemoptysis and leg pain. The most useful features for excluding PE were the absence of sudden dyspnoea, any dyspnoea and tachypnoea. Nevertheless, the authors concluded that individual features only slightly raised or lowered the probability of PE. Taken alone, they had limited diagnostic value and none ought to be used to rule in or rule out PE without further testing.

It is estimated that about 40 per cent of patients with a DVT who have no pulmonary symptoms have abnormal lung scintigrams indicating PE. Thus, much minor PE remains asymptomatic. In the 10 per cent of these patients who obstruct a branch pulmonary artery, pulmonary infarction will occur with sudden dyspnoea and usually sharp pleuritic pain associated with haemoptysis. The incidence of infarction is higher in the presence of chronic respiratory or cardiac disease. In minor embolism, there will be no central cyanosis due to relatively insignificant ventilation-perfusion mismatch and normal right ventricular function with preservation of the cardiac output.

A large clot occluding a major pulmonary artery or partially obstructing the main pulmonary artery (i.e. >50% of the pulmonary vascular bed) will result in an acute increase in right ventricular afterload and an elevation in pulmonary artery pressure, with an increased likelihood of a sudden cardiac death. The commonest clinical features in this situation are syncope (often in the context of paradoxical bradycardia), acute severe dyspnoea, acute right heart failure, cardiogenic shock and cardiac arrest with electromechanical dissociation/pulseless electrical activity. Significant cardiorespiratory compromise leads to a sinus tachycardia, tachypnoea and central cyanosis through ventilation-perfusion mismatch. To maintain cardiac output, the pulmonary artery pressure rises with consequent pressure load (up to 55 mmHg) on the right ventricle increasing right ventricular work.

In otherwise fit patients, once more than 25 per cent of the pulmonary vascular bed is occlusive, there is an increased afterload or pressure load on the right ventricle leading to an increase in right ventricular systolic pressure. With increasing pressure load, the right ventricle will dilate (against a restrictive pericardium) with the development of functional tricuspid regurgitation, an increased right atrial pressure and, ultimately, cardiogenic shock. The paradoxical movement of a pressure-loaded right ventricle leads to left ventricular diastolic dysfunction in addition to a reduction in left ventricular pre-load through a reduced transpulmonary blood flow. Echocardiography identifies these features with an increase in end-systolic and end-diastolic diameters and septal flattening in both phases of the cardiac cycle. Left ventricular end-diastolic diameter is also reduced with significant embolism.

The mechanism of hypoxaemia in massive PE is multifactorial. It occurs through significant ventilation-perfusion mismatch, and may also occur due to intrapulmonary A-V shunting through areas poorly ventilated with residual blood flow. Shunting may also occur at an atrial level where acute right heart pressures may reverse the shunt through a patent foramen ovale. Where the cardiac output is low, insufficient gas-exchange may occur in the residual areas of perfusion leading to systemic further desaturation. Hypercapnia is rare in massive PE due to tachypnoea.

Symptoms of massive PE are severe dyspnoea (not orthopnoea), syncope and low cardiac output. Angina may occur through a combination of hypoxaemia, tachycardia and hypotension. Central cyanosis and acute right heart strain ensue. It may be difficult to hear a right ventricular gallop rhythm or widely split second heart sound in the presence of significant respiratory distress.

A differential diagnosis of acute PE includes:

- acute coronary syndrome
- acute proximal aortic dissection
- acute pulmonary oedema
- acute pneumonia
- pleurisy
- acute bronchospasm
- acute exacerbations of chronic airflow limitation
- bronchogenic carcinoma
- pneumothorax
- chest wall syndrome
- fractured rib

Investigations

12-lead electrocardiography. Although 87% of patients have an abnormal ECG, these are largely non-specific and include anterior T-wave changes, ST segment abnormalities and left or right axis deviation. In the Urokinase Pulmonary Embolism Trial (UPET), 32 per cent of patients with massive PE and 26 per cent of those with massive/submassive PE had ECG signs of acute cor pulmonale such as the $S_1Q_3T_3$ pattern, right bundle branch block (RBBB), P pulmonale or right axis deviation. The ECG may be completely normal in younger, previously fit patients.

Arterial blood gases. Hypoxaemia is very common but not universally present. In one study, a PaO_2 of >11 kPa was found in 29 per cent of patients younger than 40 compared to only 3 per cent of older patients. This is true of patients without pre-existing cardiopulmonary disease.

Chest radiography. Common radiographic appearances are atelectasis, pleural effusion, infiltrates and an effusion but non-specific. Decreased vascularity is uncommon. The presence of a normal chest x-ray in the presence of hypoxaemia in the absence of an intracardiac shunt or bronchospasm is highly suggestive of PE. Signs such as focal oligaemia (Westermark sign), a peripheral wedge-shaped opacity (Hampton's hump) or an enlarged right descending pulmonary artery (Palla's sign) are often referred to, but are actually rarely seen. The value of a chest x-ray is that it allows confirmation of other pathological processes such as pneumonia, pneumothorax or rib fracture.

D-dimer. A low plasma D-dimer concentration has a 95% negative predictive accuracy. In one study of 308 patients presenting acutely with suspected PE, patients underwent assessment of clinical probability, ventilation-perfusion scan, D-dimer and lower extremity ultrasound. Of 198 patients with suspected embolism and a D-dimer level <500 µg/L, 196 were free of PE. Of course, D-dimer levels may also be raised due to co-morbid conditions which may themselves predispose to developing PE.

Computed tomography pulmonary angiography (CTPA). This technique allows rapid tomographic imaging with continuous volume acquisition during a single breath-hold; the pulmonary vasculature is visualized with a contrast dye injection. The technique is limited by poorer visualization of the peripheral areas of the upper and lower lobes. It has become the main imaging technique for the confirmation of suspected PE, with accuracy acomparable with that of invasive pulmonary angiography. In a systematic review of 15 diagnostic studies comprising 3500 patients with suspected PE, the negative predictive value of CTPA was 99.1 per cent for PE, and was 99.4 per cent for death due to PE. This modality has the greatest sensitivity for emboli in the main, lobar or segmental pulmonary arteries with a reduced sensitivity in the subsegmental branches (e.g. a pick-up rate of 25–30 per cent), although this has improved with multidetector scanners: the PIOPED II study reported a sensitivity of multidetector CT of 83 per cent and a specificity of 96 per cent. An additional advantage of spiral CT is the ability to define non-vascular structures such as lymphadenopathy, lung tumours and emphysema and other parenchymal and pleural disease.

Ventilation-perfusion (V/Q) scan. Although often used to diagnose PE, the V/Q scan is quite non-specific and is often non-diagnostic (normal or high probability in a minority of cases). In the PIOPED study, which evaluated the V/Q scan by comparison with pulmonary angiography or post-mortem, it was apparent that PE was actually present despite non-diagnostic scans in 40 per cent of cases (Table 6.2). With an increasing background of cardiorespiratory disease (particularly chronic obstructive airways disease), the V/Q scan becomes less diagnostic with an increase in intermediate-probability scans. If a ventilation scan cannot be performed, an isolated perfusion scan is useful if it is high probability, low probability, near normal or normal. In the interpretation of perfusion scans, it is imperative that one or more segmental perfusion defects are considered diagnostic of embolism.

Table 6.2 Clinical assessment and ventilation-perfusion scan probability

V/Q scan (Probability)	Clinical Probability		
	Highly likely (80–100%)	Uncertain (20–79%)	Unlikely (0–19%)
High	96%	88%	56%
Intermediate	66%	28%	16%
Low	40%	16%	4%
Near normal/normal	0	6%	2%
Total	68%	30%	9%

Pulmonary angiography. Pulmonary angiography is the invasive gold standard for diagnosing PE and was previously used where a ventilation/perfusion scan was non-diagnostic. A positive finding is an intraluminal filling defect in two views and the demonstration of an occluded pulmonary artery with or without a trailing edge. Less specific criteria are reduced perfusion, abnormal parenchymal stain and a delayed venous return. In the PIOPED study, where 1111 pulmonary angiograms were performed, 35 per cent were positive, 61 per cent were negative, with 3 per cent non-diagnostic and 1 per cent non-completion. The interobserver agreement on findings reduces as the PE becomes smaller, i.e. from lobar to segmental to subsegmental. The mortality of pulmonary angiography is 0.5 per cent with severe cardiopulmonary compromise in 0.4 per cent, and morbidity tends to be higher in critically ill patients from intensive care. This technique requires invasive expertise and has been superseded by CTPA, but may be an appropriate investigation in patients with massive PE who are candidates for percutaneous intervention (see below).

Magnetic resonance imaging. With experienced readers, the sensitivity and specificity of MRI to detect PE is 73 and 97 per cent respectively (with the potential to improve sensitivity with gadolinium injection). The technique is more rapid, less invasive and avoids standard nephrotoxic contrast compared to pulmonary angiography. However, there is a lesser evidence base for MRI than for CTPA at present but given its proven ability to detect DVT (along with lung perfusion imaging), there is an obvious appeal for a combined technique.

Lower limb evaluation. If a lung scan is non-diagnostic, evaluation of the lower extremities is an alternative means by which to assess the need for anticoagulation. With a near-normal or low-probability scan, a negative lower limb study and a low clinical suspicion, no treatment is needed. With a low-probability scan and negative leg study, but an uncertain or high clinical suspicion, the PE estimate is between 9–25 per cent. With intermediate-probability scans, but a negative leg study, either pulmonary angiography or serial non-invasive leg studies should be done, depending on the stability of the patient. In one study to evaluate the latter course, stability was defined as absence of pulmonary oedema, right ventricular failure, systolic blood pressure <90 mmHg, syncope, tachyarrhythmia, FEV_1 <1.0 l, FVC <1.5 l, PaO_2 <7 kPa and $PaCO_2$ >6 kPa. Of 627 patients with non-diagnostic lung scans and negative serial plethysmography in whom treatment was withheld, only

1.9 per cent had a venous thromboembolic complication. This compares with 0.7 per cent of untreated patients with normal lung scans and 5.5 per cent of high-probability scans who received treatment.

Echocardiography. Acute PE causes an abrupt increase in right ventricular afterload, with subsequent dilatation and hypokinesis of the right ventricle (although other causes of pulmonary hypertension may also cause this appearance). Such echocardiographic dysfunction is associated with a high risk of mortality in patients with acute PE. For example, a right to left ventricular end-diastolic diameter ratio ≥0.9 has been shown to be an independent predictor of in-hospital death even among normotensive subjects. Right ventricular failure frequently accompanies *massive* PE and correlates with larger emboli and with the recurrence of PE. Akinesis of the mid-free wall with apical sparing (McConnell's sign) may be more common in acute PE (77 per cent sensitivity, 94 per cent specificity). It should be borne in mind that the quality of the imaging will be limited by chronic airflow limitation and obesity Transoesophageal echocardiography may permit visualization of massive emboli in the proximal pulmonary arteries, which may be enhanced by contrast. An important role of echocardiography is its use to exclude alternative cases of acute cardiorespiratory compromise such as aortic dissection, acute ventricular septal rupture, large myocardial infarction and cardiac tamponade).

Troponins and brain natriuretic peptides (BNP). Simple biomarker testing has been shown to provide prognostic information. Markers indicating myocardial damage (troponins) and ventricular stretch (BNP) in response to acute pulmonary hypertension indicate worse outcomes among patients with PE. Meta-analyses show that elevated troponins are associated with increased mortality in PE, irrespective of systemic blood pressure. However, among normotensive patients, the extra risk appeared to be modest, and levels do not sufficiently distinguish high-risk, normotensive patients from lower-risk counterparts. Similarly, patients with PE and high levels of BNP or NT-pro-BNP have been shown to have a higher risk (seven-fold) of in-hospital adverse events and 30-day all-cause mortality.

In contemporary practice, the diagnosis of PE is based on validated clinical criteria combined with selective testing in view of non-specific symptoms and signs. These clinical criteria have been incorporated into scoring systems. The most commonly used system to predict clinical probability is the Wells score (see Table 6.3). The initial system has been

Table 6.3 Wells score for diagnosis of PE

Clinical variable	Score
Clinical signs and symptoms of DVT (minimum of leg swelling and pain with palpation of the deep veins)	3
PE as or more likely than an alternative diagnosis	3
Heart rate greater than 100	1.5
Immobilization or surgery in the previous 4 weeks	1.5
Previous DVT/PE	1.5
Haemoptysis	1
Malignancy (on treatment, treated in the last 6 months or palliative)	1

DVT, deep vein thrombosis; PE, pulmonary embolism. > 4, probability of PE is 'likely'. ≤4, probbility for PE is 'unlikely'. Alternatively, < 2 is low probability, moderate is 2–6 and high is > 6.

revised, resulting in assignment of different levels of probability depending on the version used.

The European Society of Cardiology algorithm for the diagnostic approach to acute PE according to the haemodynamic stability of the patient is presented in Figure 6.1.

TREATMENT OF ACUTE PULMONARY EMBOLISM

The overriding strategy in the treatment of PE is the reduction of thrombosis, i.e. both the development and propagation of venous thrombus and the fibrinolysis or break-up of established, embolized clot. With the acute presentation of a PE, it is imperative that the diagnosis is made quickly and an assessment of the patient's haemodynamic state is made. The primary therapies are:

- **Heparin**. This may be done as an initial therapy at the start of the diagnostic process.

- **Oxygen supplementation.** Initially by face mask, although supportive ventilation may be necessary. Mechanical ventilation, when needed, should be used cautiously to limit any associated adverse haemodynamic effects. For example, the increased

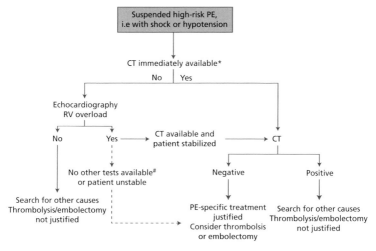

Figure 6.1 (a) Proposed algorithm for diagnosis of high-risk PE (presenting with shock/hypotension). *CT is considered not immediately available also if the critical condition of a patient allows only bedside diagnostic tests. #Transoesophageal echocardiography may detect thrombi in the pulmonary arteries in a significant proportion of patients with right ventricular overload and PE that is ultimately confirmed by CT; confirmation of DVT with bedside lower limb ultrasound might also help in decision-making.

    intrathoracic pressure induced by mechanical ventilation may reduce venous return and potentiate right ventricular dysfunction in patients with massive PE.

- **Haemodynamic support.** Noradrenaline may be used in small doses to support the acute failure of the right ventricle, but only where the patient is in cardiogenic shock as it may be counter-productive with respect to cardiac rhythm. Right heart filling pressure should be supported to maintain right ventricular stroke volume, although this is finely balanced as volume loading may exacerbate paradoxical septal motion leading to a reduction in left ventricular stroke volume. In the absence of circulatory failure, a strategy of anticoagulation is required. With haemodynamic compromise, thrombolysis and/or clot fragmentation is required.

Heparin anticoagulation

The heparin–antithrombin III complex inactivates thrombin and, to a lesser extent, activated factors IX and X. The efficacy of heparin in PE is through prevention of *further* fibrin generation from thrombin

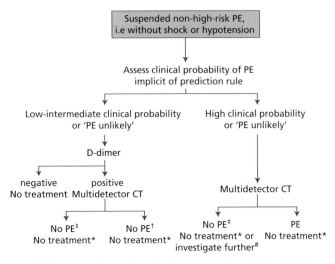

Figure 6.1 (b) Proposed algorithm for diagnosis of non-high-risk PE (presenting without shock/hypotension). *Anticoagulant treatment for PE. [†]CT is considered diagnostic of PE if the most proximol thrombus is at least segmental. [‡]If single detector CT is negative, a negative lower limb venous ultrasonography is required in order to safely exclude PE. [#]If multidetector CT is negative in patients with high clinical probability, further investigation may be considered before withholding PE-specific treatment.

Reproduced with permission from Torbicki, et al. (2008)

activation, thus allowing the endogenous fibrinolytic system to dissolve residual thrombus. Unfractionated heparin (UFH) should be given early to achieve an adequate plasma concentration, and through this and subsequent oral anticoagulation, the risk of recurrent venous thromboembolism and death is considerably reduced. By convention, UFH is given by initial bolus and intravenous infusion to achieve adequate anticoagulation. If the aPTT is prolonged prior to heparin therapy, consider antiphospholipid antibodies as a prothrombotic influence (and direct anticoagulation by the heparin level itself rather than by aPTT monitoring). Rarely, antithrombin III deficiency will lead to true heparin resistance.

The problem with UFH lies in its unpredictable haematological response due to the binding of heparin to plasma and endothelial proteins, regardless of weight adjustment. To control for this, the aPTT should also be measured 4–6 hours after initiation and similarly after any dose change to be maintained at 1.5 to 2.5 times the mean control value. Oral anticoagulation should be started simultaneously with heparin discontinued once the INR is >2.0 on two consecutive days. Serious complications from heparin therapy occur in less than 5 per cent of patients and haemorrhagic sequelae occur where there is an existing bleeding diathesis or pathology such as active or previous peptic ulcer disease/varices/angiodysplasia, recent surgery, severe hypertension or recent haemorrhagic stroke. Long-term (>2 months) heparin therapy is associated with osteoporosis and skin rashes and hypersensitivity reactions can occur. Heparin-induced thrombocytopenia (HIT) may be mild within the first few days of treatment due to direct aggregation, but if severe (<100×10^9/L), when it occurs due to antibody formation after 5–7 days, it should be discontinued with substitution by a direct antithrombin drug, e.g. hirudin or bivalirudin, as significant pro-thrombotic risk exists. This HIT with thrombosis is very serious and any potential effect of heparin on platelets should be monitored with immediate discontinuation if the platelet count drops. The direct thrombin inhibitors such as hirudin or lepirudin (recombinant hirudin) are peptides that inhibit fibrin deposition inside thrombus better than the larger heparin–antithrombin III complex giving a better inhibition to thrombus development. They have a short half-life (<2 hours) but can be monitored by the aPTT also.

Low-molecular-weight heparin

LMWH has become the treatment of choice for venous thromboembolism. It is produced by depolymerization of UFH leading to small molecules capable of inhibiting activated factor X in preference to thrombin (activated factor II). Given a longer half-life and less ancillary binding, the anticoagulant dose is predictable after subcutaneous dosing. As the aPTT measures antithrombin activity, LMWH, if necessary, should be monitored by its anti-Xa activity. Its administration subcutaneously requires less supervision and may be given once or twice daily (depending on exact LMWH type) to give as effective a therapy as UFH in the treatment of proximal DVT and acute PE. Its role in massive pulmonary embolism is less well validated, however.

The use of LMWH can be problematic and it should be given with care in patients with renal failure. Intravenous UFH, which is not renally cleared, should be the preferred mode of initial anticoagulation for patients with severe renal impairment (creatinine clearance <30 mL/min); it may also be preferable among those at high risk of bleeding, as its anticoagulant effect can be reversed quickly.

Thrombolytic therapy

Thrombolytic therapy is indicated in the treatment of massive PE (shock, severe hypoxaemia) or PE with echocardiographic right ventricular dysfunction. Because of its ability to promote fibrinolyis it has additional benefit in breaking up residual deep venous thrombus and reduces the risk of recurrent PE and chronic thromboembolism. There are several thrombolytic agents that have been used, streptokinase, urokinase, and the more fibrin-specific tissue plasminogen activator and reteplase, which work through different means to activate breakdown of plasminogen to plasmin which degrades fibrin in clot. All appear to be equally effective and safe. Thrombolysis has been shown to resolve thrombotic obstruction and to improve haemodynamic parameters. However, despite the appeal, there are few data from randomized trials of thrombolytic therapy against heparin powered to demonstrate a difference in hard clinical outcomes.

Contraindications to thrombolytic therapy are similar to those in the treatment of myocardial infarction. However, while most benefit is derived when treatment is started within 48 hours of symptom onset, thrombolysis can still be useful in patients up to 2 weeks later. Heparin should be withheld until the aPTT is less than 2:1 after thrombolysis. The risk of bleeding is greatest where the administration of thrombolysis is prolonged or where vascular puncture sites are present. If persistent major bleeding occurs, plasmin activity can be reversed by intravenous aprotinin and fibrinogen replenished with clotting factors in fresh frozen plasma (which will contain plasminogen).

Suggested doses for thrombolytic drugs for pulmonary embolism are:

- streptokinase 0.25–0.5 M over 15 minutes followed by 0.1 MU/h for 24 hours
- urokinase 4400 U/kg over 10 minutes then 4400 U/kg for 12 hours
- tPA 10 mg bolus, then 90 mg over 2 hours
- reteplase two 10 U boluses 30 minutes apart

Pulmonary embolectomy

The rapid restoration of pulmonary blood flow is likely to be a major determinant in preventing the mortality from massive PE. In the past, surgery was considered the best means of removing significant clot load. The vogue for surgical embolectomy even in extreme situations is diminishing. Historically, patients in shock despite inotropic support who continue to deteriorate and those with major contraindications to thrombolysis have been considered for surgical embolectomy. Retrospective series largely pre-date the use of thrombolysis and include procedures outside the emergency setting. High operative mortality of up to 50 per cent has been reported, and current practice has included femoral-to-femoral bypass for haemodynamic support prior to full cardiopulmonary bypass. The need for cardiopulmonary resuscitation prior to surgery predicts an adverse outcome from surgical embolectomy. With survival from the procedure, most late morbidity is neurological.

Mechanical thrombectomy

In the modern era of percutaneous intervention, attempts have been made to provide an alternative to surgical embolectomy. Initial techniques have focused on retrieval devices to hold and extract a thrombus from the main pulmonary artery in patients with massive PE. However, this approach has been of limited success. Clot fragmentation has been described in uncontrolled studies using a pigtail catheter. The theoretical benefit of this approach is that the clot will fragment into a smaller vascular area as it embolizes distally and will be more susceptible to thrombolysis. This will reduce pulmonary artery pressure and improve transpulmonary flow in most cases. In cases where pulmonary artery pressure remains high, this may occur through release of vasoconstrictor hormones such as thromboxane A_2 arguing for the actual removal of clot rather than simple embolization of it. Again, outcome data for this technique are limited. However, newer devices are becoming available which both fragment and aspirate clots such as the Hydrolyser™, Amplatz™ and Günther catheters. The most promising device may be the Arrow-Trerotola percutaneous thrombolytic device (PTD), which consists of a motor-driven 5F outer catheter connected to a fragmentation basket which rotates at 3000 rpm. The latest version of this device may be introduced over-the-wire through a guide catheter into the thrombus and activated to fragment the thrombus.

Clinical studies are also ongoing with respect to the fragmentation of ileofemoral thrombus via the transjugular route using this device. It can be deployed in the pelvic veins with the adjunctive use of a temporarily deployed wallstent in the inferior vena cavae to act as a filter for old thrombus which can then be removed back into a large 15F guide catheter.

Chronic treatment of acute pulmonary embolism
Oral anticoagulation
It is imperative that warfarin is started after diagnosis is made and acute treatment started so that an overlap can occur for a 5-day period to avoid

the pro-thrombotic state created by a reduction in protein C with oral anticoagulation. The prothrombin time expressed as the INR should be adjusted to a therapeutic window of 2.0–3.0, or higher where the antiphospholipid syndrome is the cause of the thromboembolism. In the medium-term treatment of the patient, obvious risk factors should be corrected which may allow a shorter period of anticoagulation compared to the standard period of 3 months for a first PE. In the presence of a persistent procoagulant stimulus such as malignant disease or proven thrombophilia or where recurrent PE has occurred (prior PE is the best predictor of recurrent DVT) or where the patient has chronic thromboembolic disease, treatment should be prolonged or lifelong. Significant bleeding complications with over-anticoagulation should be treated with a bolus of 0.5–1.0 mg of vitamin K that will bring the INR back into the normal range. This can take up to 24 hours so clotting factor concentrates or fresh frozen plasma should be given for quicker restoration of haemostasis.

Anticoagulation is required to reduce the risk of proximal propagation and embolism to the pulmonary circulation. DVT proximal to the calf and symptomatic calf (popliteal) DVTs require LMWH injections and an arbitrary 3-month course of warfarin. A 20 per cent recurrence rate has been reported in the literature. Patients with symptomatic DVT do not all require hospital admission and patients may be risk stratified according to PE risk (see Table 6.1). Long-term anticoagulation is required in significantly obese patients and in those with cancer and previous DVT. Anticoagulation is not mandatory in asymptomatic calf DVTs as long as serial ultrasound monitoring confirms no proximal extension. A majority of patients develop chronic venous insufficiency after anticoagulant therapy and the use of high-pressure support stockings prevent venous wall distension on ambulation, which may reduce this risk.

Inferior vena caval filters

These filters can be introduced, delivered and deployed percutaneously to prevent significant thrombus reaching the pulmonary circulation. Their use should be restricted to situations where recurrent DVTs occur despite adequate anticoagulation or used in patients who cannot tolerate warfarin on a temporary or permanent basis. The long-term outcome of these devices is less good with caval thrombosis at the filter site, filter fracture and migration and occasional vessel wall perforation.

Thromboembolic pulmonary disease

Patients with recurrent PE may go on to develop chronic thromboembolic disease with pulmonary hypertension and ultimately cor pulmonale. This occurs where recurrent PE has been undiagnosed over several weeks to months without oral anticoagulation. The best treatment option for this rare condition is surgical thromboendarterectomy with removal of organized clot ideally as a cast of the pulmonary vascular tree. As with acute surgical embolectomy, this operation carries a significant mortality and it is likely that a percutaneous thrombectomy technique will supersede this approach in the future.

KEY POINTS

- PE occurs through dislodgment of a venous thrombus from the deep leg or the pelvic veins into the pulmonary arterial circulation. The clinical signs of embolism are determined by the level at which the thrombus is occlusive.

- The development of a venous thrombus is determined by Virchow's triad of local injury, hypercoagulability and stasis of flow.

- Venous thromboembolism is a clinical situation where the diagnosis is more often not made than made. The clinical suspicion of a DVT (leg swelling, calf tenderness, venous distension of subcutaneous vessels, discolouration) should be confirmed objectively, due to the lack of predictive accuracy in the clinical examination.

- In the presence of a suspected acute DVT, either compression ultrasound or impedance plethysmography should be done. If inconclusive or inadequate, venography or MRI should be done.

- In acute PE, classic symptoms are unexplained dyspnoea, pleuritic chest pain and haemoptysis with tachypnoea in particular and tachycardia being common signs, but all are non-specific.

- The V/Q scan is often non-specific and in one study which evaluated the V/Q scan by pulmonary angiography or post-mortem, it was apparent that PE was often present in the presence of non-diagnostic scans in 40 per cent of cases.

- CTPA is limited by poorer visualization of the peripheral areas of the lung but is associated with 95 per cent specificity and sensitivity for PE. CTPA has the greatest sensitivity for emboli in the main, lobar or segmental pulmonary arteries.

- The treatment of acute PE includes intravenous heparin, oxygen supplementation and haemodynamic support with noradrenaline and careful volume balance. In the absence of circulatory failure, a strategy of anticoagulation is required. With haemodynamic compromise, thrombolysis and/or clot fragmentation is required.

- Clinical studies are ongoing with the percutaneous use of a thrombolytic device which consists of a motor-driven catheter connected to a fragmentation basket rotating at high speed. Other percutaneous devices use the Venturi effect to aspirate fresh clot both in the deep venous system and in the pulmonary circulation.

KEY REFERENCES

Brady AJB, Crake T, Oakley CM. Percutaneous catheter fragmentation and distal dispersion of proximal pulmonary embolus. *Lancet* 1991; **338**: 1186–9.

Fava M, Loyola S, Flores P, Huete I. Mechanical fragmentation and pharmacologic thrombolysis in massive pulmonary embolism. *J Vasc Intervent Radiol* 1997; **8**: 261–6.

Goldhaber SZ, Markis JE, Meyerovitz MF, et al. Acute pulmonary embolism treated with tissue plasminogen activator. *Lancet* 1986; **18**: 886–9.

Green RM, Meyer TJ, Dunn M, Glassroth J. Pulmonary embolism in younger adults. *Chest* 1992; **101**: 1507–11.

Greenfield LJ, Proctor MC, Williams DM, Wakefield TW. Long-term experience with transvenous catheter pulmonary embolectomy. *J Vasc Surg* 1993; **18**: 450–8.

Hirsh J, Dalen JE, Anderson DR, et al. Oral anticoagulants: mechanism of action, clinical effectiveness, and optimal therapeutic range. *Chest* 1998; **114**: 445S–69S.

Hull RD, Raskob G, Ginsberg JS, Panju A, Brill-Edwards P, Caotes G, Pineo GF. A noninvasive strategy for the treatment of patients with suspected pulmonary embolism. *Arch Intern Med* 1994; **154**: 289–97.

Konstantinides SV. Acute pulmonary embolism revisited. *Heart* 2008; **94**: 795–802.

Leclerc JR, Illescas F, Jarzem P. Diagnosis of deep vein thrombosis. In: Leclerc JR (ed), *Venous Thromboembolic Disorders*. Philadelphia: Lea & Febiger 1991; 176–228.

McConnell MV, Solomon SD, Rayan ME, Come PC, Goldhaber SZ, Lee RT. Regional right ventricular dysfunction detected by echocardiography in acute pulmonary embolism. *Am. J. Cardiol* 1996; **78**(4): 469–73.

Moser KM, Daily PO, Peterson K, et al. Thromboendarterectomy for chronic major-vessel thromboembolic pulmonary hypertension; immediate and long-term results in 42 patients. *Ann Intern Med* 1987; **107**: 560.

Perrier A, Bounameaux H, Morabia A, et al. Diagnosis of pulmonary embolism by a decision analysis-based strategy including clinical probability, D-dimer levels, and ultrasonography: a management study. *Arch Intern Med* 1996; **156**: 531–6.

Piazza G, Goldhaber SZ. Acute pulmonary embolism. Part I: epidemiology and diagnosis. *Circulation* 2006; **114**: e28–32.

Piazza G, Goldhaber SZ. Acute pulmonary embolism. Part II: treatment and prophylaxis. *Circulation* 2006; **114**: e42–e47.

PIOPED investigators. Value of the ventilation-perfusion scan in acute pulmonary embolism: results of the Prospective Investigation of Pulmonary Embolism Diagnosis (PIOPED). *JAMA* 1990; **263**: 2753–9.

Ricek M, Peregrin J, Velimsky T. Mechanical thrombectomy of massive pulmonary embolism using an Arrow-Trerotola percutaneous thrombolytic device. *Eur Radiol* 1998; **8**: 163–5.

Riedel M. Therapy of pulmonary thromboembolism, Part 1: acute massive pulmonary embolism. *Cor vasa* 1996; **38**: 93–102.

Sanchez O, Planquette B, Meyer G. Update on acute pulmonary embolism. *ERR* 2009; **18**: 137–47.

Stein PD, Fowler SE, Goodman LR, et al. Multidetector computed tomography for acute pulmonary embolism. *N Engl J Med* 2006; **354**: 2317–27.

Torbicki A, Perrier A, Konstantinides S, et al. Guidelines on the diagnosis and management of acute pulmonary embolism: the Task Force for the Diagnosis and Management of Acute Pulmonary Embolism of the European Society of Cardiology (ESC). *Eur Heart J* 2008; **29**: 2276–315.

Urokinase Pulmonary Embolism Trial: a national co-operative study. *Circulation* 1973; **47**(Suppl.II): I–108.

Verstraete M, Miller GAH, Bounameaux H, et al. Intravenous and intrapulmonary recombinant tissue-type plasminogen activator in the treatment of acute massive pulmonary embolism. *Circulation* 1988; **77**: 353–60.

Wells PS. Integrated strategies for the diagnosis of venous thromboembolism. *J Thromb Haemost* 2007; **5**(suppl): 41–50.

West J, Goodacre S, Sampson F. The value of clinical features in the diagnosis of acute pulmonary embolism: systematic review and meta-analysis. *QJM* 2007; **100**: 763–9.

INFECTIVE ENDOCARDITIS

BACKGROUND

Epidemiology and pathophysiology

Strictly speaking, infective endocarditis (IE) is a disease in which an infective organism colonizes the heart valves, septal defects or mural endocardium. However, in clinical practice the definition extends to include infections on arteriovenous shunts, arterio-arterial shunts and aortic coarctations, as the clinical presentation is often indistinguishable. The infection evolves to produce a vegetation that comprises an amorphous mass of organisms, inflammatory cells, fibrin and platelets. Following successful treatment for IE, healing occurs by fibrosis and calcification.

Overall, there are approximately 1500 cases of endocarditis in the UK per year, with an estimated in-patient mortality between 15 and 20 per cent. IE can occur not only on congenital or acquired structural cardiac abnormalities but also on normal, previously healthy valves. Traditionally, endocarditis has been divided into acute and subacute forms. Acute bacterial endocarditis is usually due to a virulent organism such as *Staphylococcus aureus*, which can rapidly lead to complications within days or weeks if left untreated. Subacute bacterial endocarditis is more indolent, usually presents weeks to months after the initial infection and is caused by organisms such as *Streptococcus viridans* or coagulase-negative staphylococci. This classification was initially based on untreated disease. Since devastating complications such as valve perforation and cerebral embolization arise with a variety of different organisms and bacteria are not always implicated, the term IE is more appropriate and is now widely used.

In the past, IE occurred mainly in patients with underlying rheumatic or congenital heart disease. The incidence and prevalence of rheumatic heart disease has decreased in developed countries. Contemporary causes of IE affecting the native valves include mitral valve prolapse (accounting for up to one-third of cases in adults), bicuspid aortic valves, degenerative/sclerotic valves (particularly in an ageing population) and intravenous drug use (IVDU). IE associated with IVDU is usually associated with right-sided valve lesions, and can affect up to 7 per cent of subjects with previous IVDU. In the United States, up to 12 per cent of acute drug-related presentations relate to IE. *Staphylococcus aureus* is responsible for more than 50 per cent of these infections. Unusual organisms such as *Corynebacterium* species, *Bacillus cereus*, *Lactobacillus*, *Candida* and polymicrobial infections can sometimes be found in this population. In addition, it is now recognized that many older patients are developing IE as a result of invasive procedures and nosocomial infections. Congenital heart disease is more important as a cause of IE in young adults.

In developed countries, epidemiological studies suggest that 10–20 per cent of patients with prosthetic heart valves develop endocarditis. The risk is greatest during the first 6 months after valve surgery and thereafter declines to about 0.2–0.35 per cent per year. The term 'early' is often used to describe prosthetic valve endocarditis when it occurs within 2 months following surgery, when it is considered to be a complication of valve surgery. Prosthetic valve endocarditis occurring more than 12 months after surgery is termed 'late' and, like native valve endocarditis, is likely to be associated with community-acquired infections. Cases occurring between 2 and 12 months after surgery are a mixture of hospital-acquired episodes caused by less virulent organisms and community-acquired episodes. Hence, the timing of infection reflects different pathogenic mechanisms, which in turn influence the epidemiology, microbiology, pathology and clinical manifestation. The risk of invasive infection is increased among patients with prosthetic valve endocarditis within the first year after implantation, particularly those with infection of an aortic valve prosthesis. Table 7.1 summarizes the microbiology of IE in native and prosthetic heart valves, and in subjects with a history of IVDU.

The pathogenesis of IE involves turbulent blood flow from a high to a low pressure zone, resulting in damage and ulceration to the endocardium. The contact between blood and the subendothelial surfaces promotes production of thrombus. Micro-organisms present in the blood may then

Table 7.1 Microbiology of infective endocarditis

Organism	Non-addicts (per cent)	Addicts (per cent)	Early PVE (per cent)	Late PVE (per cent)
Streptococcus viridans	50	10	8	30
Enterococci	5	8	2	6
Other streptococci	5	2		
Staphylococcus aureus	20	57	15	10
Staphylococcus epidermidis	5	3	33	29
Gram-negative bacteria (including HACEK group)[a]	6	7	17	10
Fungus	1	5	10	5
Culture negative	5	5	5	5
Diphtheroids			8	3
Mixed/Others	3	3	2	2

[a]The HACEK group of organisms consists of *Haemophilus* species, *Actinobacillus* species, *Cardiobacterium* species, *Eikenella* species and *Kingella* species. These Gram-negative coccobacilli are fastidious and slow growing, and have become an important cause of IE. They are part of the respiratory tract and oropharyngeal flora.

seed to the thrombus and proliferate, resulting in IE. In addition, *Staphylococcus aureus* possesses binding proteins on its surface, which facilitates adhesion to focal areas of local inflammation that are rich in fibronectin. Vegetations are usually located along the line of closure of a valve leaflet on the low pressure side of the valve where turbulence occurs (i.e. the atrial surface for atrioventricular valves or the ventricular surface for semilunar valves). The absence of a pressure gradient across an ostium secundum atrial septal defect explains the low risk of endocarditis in this group.

CLINICAL PRESENTATION

The clinical syndrome of IE consists of fever, changing murmurs, septic embolization to any organ and petechial lesions of the skin. The diagnosis should be suspected in anyone who presents with pyrexia and multisystem involvement in the presence of cardiac disease or prior IVDU.

Acute IE presentations are usually characterized by a toxic, unwell patient with high fevers and rigors. Subacute or chronic presentations often occur weeks or months after the initial infection, and can be associated with a low-grade fever, night sweats, weight loss and anaemia (normochromic normocytic). Other associated symptoms and signs may include lethargy, anorexia, vague abdominal or flank pain, confusion, arthralgia, myalgia and finger clubbing. Peripheral manifestations as a result of an immunologically mediated vasculitis or septic embolization can give rise to:

- Osler's nodes (tender, subcutaneous nodules seen in the pulps of the digits);
- Janeway lesions (non-tender, erythematous or haemorrhagic macular lesions seen on the palms and soles);
- splinter haemorrhages in the fingernails or toenails; petechiae on the conjunctivae and buccal mucosa;
- focal glomerulonephritis and splenic infarcts;
- mycotic aneurysms and occlusion involving any vessel, commonly seen in the cerebral arteries, abdominal aorta, coronary arteries, gastrointestinal arteries, limb arteries and renal arterioles;
- retinal infarcts (Roth's spots), causing an oval-shaped haemorrhage with a pale centre;
- neurological involvement in 30–40 per cent of patients with IE, the majority of which are embolic strokes, with intracranial haemorrhages occurring in 5 per cent;
- congestive cardiac failure as a result of valve destruction or rupture of a chorda and, rarely, intracardiac fistulae, myocarditis or coronary artery embolism;
- perivalvular extension beyond the valve ring either in native or prosthetic valve IE, giving rise to paravalvular regurgitation, valve dehiscence, septal and myocardial abscesses, fistulous tracts, pericarditis and conduction disturbances such as first degree AV block;
- a change in the quality of the audible prosthetic clicks can reflect valve obstruction by vegetation overgrowth.

Because patients with prosthetic heart valves are always at risk for IE, the presence of fever or new prosthesis dysfunction at any time warrants consideration of the diagnosis.

Heart murmurs are heard in 80–85 per cent of patients with IE but may be difficult to detect or be absent in patients with tricuspid valve involvement. Careful auscultation in full inspiration is often useful in diagnosing right-sided murmurs. Septic pulmonary embolization from right-sided valvular IE (frequently seen in IVDU-related IE) can give rise to shortness of breath, haemoptysis, pleuritic chest pain and pulmonary abscesses.

Poor prognostic factors include increased age, infection of a prosthetic valve, patients with cardiac complications on admission, persistent sepsis, type of organism involved (*Staphylococcus*, fungal and nosocomial infections carry a higher risk than *Streptococcus viridans* infection), and the presence of associated diseases such as chronic renal disease, chronic liver disease, neoplasms and HIV.

DIAGNOSIS AND INVESTIGATIONS

IE is largely a *clinical* diagnosis, based on history and clinical examination, that is confirmed with blood cultures and echocardiography. It is important to search for a portal of entry of infection, which may give a clue to the type of organism causing the infection. For instance, *Streptococcus viridans* infections frequently occur following dental procedures or poor oral hygiene, enterococcal infections occur after genitourinary and gastrointestinal procedures or in women after abortion or giving birth, and staphylococcal, Gram-negative bacterial and fungal infections in drug abusers and after open heart surgery. Alternatively, the causative organism may be associated with an underlying condition, for instance *Streptococcus bovis* IE is frequently associated with colonic polyps and cancer. Most cases of procedure-related IE occur with a short incubation period of approximately 2 weeks or less following the procedure.

The variability in the clinical presentation of IE requires a diagnostic strategy that is sensitive for disease detection and specific for its exclusion. Use of the Duke criteria (developed at Duke University, United States in 1994) is currently recommended by the American College of Cardiology/American Heart Association (ACC/AHA) and has been adopted internationally to aid the diagnosis of IE. A definite diagnosis of IE can be made either pathologically or clinically. A pathological diagnosis is made when pathological specimens from surgery or autopsy reveal positive histology or culture. A clinical diagnosis is made by determining the presence of major and/or minor criteria as seen in Box 7.1. A diagnosis of IE is made if there are two major or one major and three minor or five minor criteria.

Blood cultures are paramount for diagnosis and monitoring treatment. Three sets of cultures (aerobic and anaerobic) containing at least 10 mL

Box 7.1 Definitions of terms used in the modified Duke criteria for the diagnosis of IE[a]

Major criteria

Positive blood culture for IE

Typical micro-organism consistent with IE from 2 separate blood cultures as noted below:
- (1) viridans streptococci, *Streptococcus bovis*, HACEK group, *Staphylococcus aureus* or
- (2) community-acquired enterococci in the absence of a primary focus, or

micro-organisms consistent with IE from persistently positive blood cultures defined as:
- (1) >2 positive cultures of blood samples drawn >12 hours apart or
- (2) all of 3 or a majority of >4 separate cultures of blood (with first and last sample drawn >1 hour apart).

Positive blood culture for *Coxiella burnetii* or antiphase 1 IgG antibody titre .1:800.

Evidence of endocardial involvement

Positive echocardiogram for IE defined as:
- (1) oscillating intracardiac mass on valve or supporting structures, in the path of regurgitant jets, or on implanted material in the absence of an alternative anatomical explanation, or
- (2) abscess, or
- (3) new partial dehiscence of prosthetic valve, or new valvular regurgitation (worsening or changing of pre-existing murmur not sufficient).

Note: TOE is recommended in patients with prosthetic valves who are rated as having at least possible IE by clinical criteria, or who have complicated IE such as paravalvular abscesses, etc.

Continued

Minor criteria

(1) Predisposition: predisposing heart condition or intravenous drug use

(2) Fever: temperature >38.0°C

(3) Vascular phenomena: major arterial emboli, septic pulmonary infarcts, mycotic aneurysm, intracranial haemorrhage, conjunctival haemorrhages, and Janeway lesions

(4) Immunological phenomena: glomerulonephritis, Osler's nodes, Roth spots, and rheumatoid factor

(5) Microbiological evidence: positive blood culture but does not meet a major criterion as noted above or serological evidence of active infection with organism consistent with IE

---

[a]A diagnosis of IE is made if there are two major or one major and three minor or five minor criteria. Possible IE is suspected if there is one major and one minor criterion, or three minor criteria.

Adapted from Li, et al. *Clin Infect Dis* 2000; **30**: 633–8.

of blood should be taken from different sites, at different times (30–60-minute intervals), and before commencement of antibiotics. Blood cultures are negative in ≤5 per cent of patients with IE diagnosed by strict diagnostic criteria. Negative blood cultures may occur as a result of inadequate microbiological techniques, infection with highly fastidious bacteria or non-bacterial organisms, or administration of antibiotics prior to obtaining blood cultures. Specialized microbiological techniques and culture media, prolonged incubation periods as well as serology (for organisms such as *Brucella*, *Legionella*, *Bartonella*, *Coxiella burnetii* or *Chlamydia* species) may be needed to diagnose unusual organisms. The use of blood tests for polymerase chain reaction (PCR) may also become more widely used in difficult to culture organisms. Swabs should be taken from skin lesions, cannulation sites and the nasal cavity. Early and close liaison with the microbiology department is essential.

Echocardiography is not an appropriate screening test in the evaluation of patients with fever or a positive blood culture that is unlikely to reflect IE. Nevertheless, echocardiography should be performed in all patients suspected of having IE clinically. An observational study of

500 patients with suspected endocarditis assessed whether clinical features could guide decisions to use transthoracic echocardiography. The collective absence of the following five clinical factors was associated with a zero probability of the transthoracic echocardiography showing evidence of endocarditis. These factors are in descending order of risk:

- vasculitic or embolic phenomena
- the presence of central venous access
- a recent history of injected drug use
- the presence of a prosthetic valve
- positive blood cultures.

Transthoracic echocardiography is readily available, non-invasive and has a sensitivity of <60 per cent for vegetations <2 mm and a specificity of 98 per cent. In patients in whom IE or its complications are strongly suspected, a negative transthoracic echo will not definitely rule out IE and transoesophageal echocardiography (TOE) is recommended. TOE has a sensitivity of 76–100 per cent and a specificity of 94 per cent. It can diagnose vegetations <1 mm and is useful in evaluating and monitoring patients who develop complications and in patients with a suspected diagnosis of prosthetic valve endocarditis (compared to transthoracic echocardiography, TOE allows better visualization of prosthetic valves).

Haematological indices are frequently abnormal and include a raised erythrocyte sedimentation rate (ESR), leucocytosis, normochromic normocytic anaemia, low serum iron and a low serum iron binding capacity. Findings of immune stimulation and ongoing inflammation include a raised C-reactive protein (CRP), rheumatoid factor, hypocomplementaemia (decreased C3/C4) and cryoglobulinaemia. Urine analysis may show haematuria, red cell casts and proteinuria as a result of glomerular involvement. Although there may be no specific changes on the ECG, the development of PR interval prolongation may signify the presence of an aortic root or septal abscess. Chest x-ray may show signs of heart failure and pulmonary infiltrates from septic emboli.

It is important to recognize that the majority of symptoms, signs and laboratory investigations seen in IE are not specific and can also occur in other diseases such as connective tissue disorders, atrial myxoma, acute rheumatic fever and lymphomas.

ANTIMICROBIAL TREATMENT AND MONITORING

If the diagnosis is suspected and cultures have been taken, then IV antibiotics should be commenced. The choice of agents used for empirical treatment has changed over the years with the change in incidence of endocarditis due to *Staphylococcus aureus*. The Working Party of the British Society for Antimicrobial Chemotherapy recommend empirical treatment based on presentation:

Acute presentation	Flucloxacillin (8–12 g IV daily in 4–6 divided doses) plus gentamicin (1 mg/kg IV 8 hourly, modified according to renal function)
Indolent presentation	Penicillin (7.2 g IV daily in 6 divided doses) or ampicillin/amoxycillin (2 g IV 6 hourly) plus gentamicin (1 mg/kg IV 8 hourly, modified according to renal function)
Penicillin allergy or intracardiac prosthesis or suspected MRSA	Vancomycin (1 g 12 hourly IV, modified according to renal function) plus rifampicin (300–600 mg 12 hourly by mouth) plus gentamicin (1 mg/kg IV 8 hourly, modified according to renal function)

The choice and duration of antimicrobial therapy for patients with IE should eventually be dictated by the pathogens identified from blood cultures. Full discussion of the specific therapeutic regimens is beyond the scope of this chapter and should be decided upon in collaboration with the microbiologists. Close collaboration with the microbiologist is essential, in particular when blood cultures are negative in order to avoid inappropriate treatment and to discuss alternative investigation.

Most patients with IE respond to appropriate antibiotic treatment within 72 hours, with a reduction in fever and improvement in general well-being. If fever persists or recurs, then further blood cultures should be taken. The recurrence of fever during treatment does not necessarily indicate an unsatisfactory response to antibiotics, but may indicate a hypersensitivity reaction to drugs, phlebitis, an infection elsewhere or major immune activation (Table 7.2). Urine analysis should be done daily, ECGs should be obtained twice weekly and echocardiography weekly. A falling CRP and ESR are reassuring.

Table 7.2 Some causes of persistent or recurrent fever during treatment of infective endocarditis

---

Infection related

Intracardiac: Paravalvular/intracardiac abscesses

Extracardiac: Line infection, metastatic infection, mycotic aneurysms, spinal abscess, vertebral osteomyelitis, discitis, etc.

Antibiotic resistance: seldom a cause especially if the infecting bacteria has been cultured and sensitivity determined

Antibiotic sensitivity

Can be associated with or without a rash, eosinophilia and a rise in CRP in a patient who had been previously doing well

Major immune activation

Associated with progressive renal failure, vasculitis, emboli, etc.

Multiple organisms

Usually seen in intravenous drug abusers

Wrong diagnosis

Lymphoma, sarcoidosis, AIDS, tuberculosis, atrial myxoma, acute rheumatic fever, autoimmune disease such as SLE, etc.

ANTICOAGULANT THERAPY

Anticoagulant therapy has not been shown to prevent embolization in IE and may increase the risk of intracerebral haemorrhage. Patients with prosthetic valve endocarditis who are receiving chronic anticoagulant therapy should be allowed to cautiously continue. However, in the presence of cerebral emboli with haemorrhage, temporary discontinuation of anticoagulation is appropriate. In unstable patients or in those for whom surgery is planned, warfarin can be discontinued and replaced with unfractionated heparin, which can easily be reversed.

COMPLICATIONS AND INDICATIONS FOR SURGERY

Patients should be seen and examined daily to screen for the development of aforementioned complications. Among the complications, heart failure has the greatest impact on prognosis. Heart failure is more frequently seen with aortic valve infections (29 per cent) than with mitral (20 per cent) or tricuspid (8 per cent) disease. The early onset of heart failure signifies the need for surgical intervention. Delaying surgery to the point of marked ventricular decompensation can dramatically increase operative mortality, from 6–11 per cent for stable patients to 17–33 per cent for patients with heart failure. The incidence of reinfection of the newly implanted valve in patients with active IE has been estimated to be 2–3 per cent, which is far less than the operative mortality rate. Therefore, surgery should never be delayed to prolong pre-operative antibiotic treatment. Other indicators for acute surgical intervention also include intracardiac abscesses and fistulous tracts, unstable valve prosthesis, persistent bacteraemia despite antimicrobial therapy, fungal infections, recurrent systemic embolization (>2 major embolic events) and large obstructive vegetations (>10 mm) (see Table 7.3). The duration of antibiotic therapy following surgery is dependent on the antibiotic

Table 7.3 IE and indications for surgery

Absolute	Relative
• Moderate to severe congestive heart failure due to valve	• Congestive heart failure resolved with medical therapy dysfunction
• Refractory infection (persistent bacteraemia, relapse after optimal therapy – prosthetic valves) with lack of improvement after more than 1 week of antibiotics	• Relapse after optimal therapy (native valves)
• Fungal infection	• Culture-negative endocarditis with persistent unexplained fever
• Unstable valve prosthesis	• Vegetations >10 mm
• Significant dehiscence of prosthetic valves	• New regurgitation in an aortic prosthesis
• Perivalvular extension with septal and myocardial abscesses, fistulous tracts, atrioventricular block, rupture of sinus of Valsalva aneurysm, rupture of subaortic aneurysm	• Single systemic embolic event
• Large vegetation causing obstruction	

• Recurrent systemic emboli
  – several episodes
  – one episode with residual large vegetation	

sensitivity of the organism, the presence of paravalvular invasive infection and the culture status of the vegetation. Generally, in endocarditis caused by antibiotic-sensitive organisms with negative cultures of operative specimens, pre-operative plus post-operative therapy should at least equal a full course of recommended therapy. Patients with positive intraoperative cultures and prosthetic valve endocarditis should receive a full course of antimicrobial therapy post-operatively.

PREVENTION

IE is a life-threatening disease and carries a high risk of morbidity and mortality despite modern antimicrobial and surgical treatment. It is therefore imperative, whenever possible, to try to prevent unnecessary infections, especially those in high-risk groups. When determining which patients need antibiotic cover, it is important to consider the underlying cardiac condition (as some conditions are more often associated with endocarditis than others), the risk of bacteraemia associated with the particular procedure, and the likely organism that may propagate to give rise to IE. Currently there is considerable controversy over when antibiotic prophylaxis should be given. Recently several guidelines advising on antibiotic prophylaxis have changed, reflecting the lack of evidence that exists for the benefits of chemoprohylaxis. Additionally, there is evidence to suggest that bacteraemia occurs with everyday activities such as chewing or brushing teeth. Consequently, in the UK, the National Institute for Health and Clinical Excellence (NICE) has published guidelines stating that prophylaxis is *not* required, except where there is evidence of active infection. This is at odds with recommendations of the AHA and ESC. The Working Party of the British Society for Antimicrobial Chemotherapy (BSAC) guidelines are similar to that of the AHA and ESC and are stated below. They recommend prophylaxis for dental procedures (involving dento-gingival manipulation) in those at high risk of endocarditis such as patients with:

- previous IE
- cardiac valve replacement
- surgically constructed systemic or pulmonary shunt or conduit.

These patients should be given amoxycillin 3 g po, 1 hour prior to the procedure. Those allergic to penicillin should be given clindamycin 600 mg po.

In addition to the above high-risk group, for non-dental procedures BSAC also defines the following groups as high risk:

- complex congenital heart disease (except secundum atrial septal defects)
- complex left ventricular outflow abnormalities, including aortic stenosis and bicuspid aortic valve
- aquired valvulopathy and mitral valve prolapse (with echocardiographic evidence of substantial leaflet abnormality and regurgitation).

For gastrointestinal diagnostic procedures, such as upper and lower gastrointestinal endoscopy, routine use of prophylaxis is not recommended except for high-risk patients as above. Prophylaxis is, however, recommended for therapeutic procedures such as ERCP or oesophageal dilatation and laser probe treatment. In the case of genitourinary procedures such as cystoscopy, urethral dilatation, transurethral resection of prostate and transrectal prostatic biopsy, antibiotic prophylaxis is recommended. For urethral catheterization routine prophylaxis is not recommended; however, antibiotics should be given if there is evidence of a urinary infection prior to catheterization. In obstetric and gynaecology procedure, antibiotics are recommended for vaginal hysterectomy and caesarian section. They are not recommended in vaginal delivery unless there is infection or prolonged rupture of the membranes, in which case antibiotics are indicated regardless of the endocarditis risk. For these non-dental procedures a single dose of amoxicillin 1 g IV (Teicoplanin 400 mg IV if penicillin allergic) and gentamicin 1 g/kg is recommended just prior to the procedure or with induction of anaesthesia.

Prophylaxis is also advised in surgery involving the upper respiratory tract, nasal packing/intubation (Flucloxacillin 1 g IV or clindamycin 600 mg IV if penicillin allergic) and for cosmetic piercing of the tongue or oral mucosa (as per dental prophylaxis). It is not recommended for bronchoscopy.

KEY POINTS

- IE is a challenging medical disease, which requires a high index of suspicion, and early diagnosis and treatment in order to be successfully managed.

- IE can involve multiple systems and can often present in a similar way to other conditions such as connective tissue disorders, atrial myxoma and lymphomas, and is therefore a great mimicker.

- Although the number of cases of IE related to rheumatic heart disease has decreased, this reduction has been balanced by an increased incidence of IE in IV drug abusers and the elderly.

- Advances in microbiology techniques and echocardiographic imaging (in particular, TOE) have improved the ability to diagnose IE.

- A multidisciplinary approach is necessary for decision-making during treatment, with consultation from cardiology, cardiothoracic surgery and the microbiology departments.

- Patients with signs and symptoms of heart failure should be considered for early surgical intervention.

- Administration of antibiotic prophylaxis is determined by the underlying cardiac condition as some conditions are more often associated with endocarditis than others, the risk of bacteraemia associated with the particular procedure, and the likely organism that may propagate to give rise to IE.

KEY REFERENCES

AHA Scientific Statement. Infective endocarditis diagnosis, antimicrobial therapy, and management of complications. *Circulation* 2005; **111**: e394–e433.

Dajani AS, Taubert KA, Wilson W, et al. Prevention of bacterial endocarditis. Recommendations by the American Heart Association. *JAMA* 1997; **277**: 1794–801.

Durack DT. Prevention of infective endocarditis. *N Engl J Med* 1995; **332**: 38–44.

Durack DT, Lukes AS, Bright DK. New criteria for the diagnosis of infective endocarditis: utilization of specific echocardiographic findings. *Am J Med* 1994; **96**: 200–9.

Greaves K, Mou D, Patel A, Celermajer D S. Clinical criteria and the appropriate use of transthoracic echocardiography for the exclusion of infective endocarditis. *Heart* 2003; **89**: 273–5.

Guidelines for the antibiotic treatment of endocarditis in adults: report of the Working Party of the British Society for Antimicrobial Chemotherapy. *J Antimicrob Chemother* 2004; **54**: 971–81.

Guidelines for the prevention of endocarditis: report of the Working Party of the British Society for Antimicrobial Chemotherapy. *J Antimicrob Chemother* 2006; **57**: 1035–42.

Li JS, Sexton DJ, Mick N, et al. Proposed modifications to the duke criteria for the diagnosis of infective endocarditis. *Clin Infect Dis* 2000; **30**: 633–8.

Mylonakis E, Calderwood SB. Infective endocarditis in adults. *N Engl J Med* 2001; **345**: 1318–30.

Oakley CM, Hall RJC. Endocarditis problems – patients being treated for endocarditis and not doing well. *Heart* 2001; **85**: 470–4.

Piper C, Korfer R, Horstotte D. Prosthetic valve endocarditis. *Heart* 2001; **85**: 590–3.

Prophylaxis against infective endocarditis – Antimicrobial prophylaxis against infective endocarditis in adults and children undergoing interventional procedures. National Institute for Health and Clinical Excellence. March 2008.

CHAPTER 8

DRUG-RELATED CARDIAC PROBLEMS

DIGOXIN TOXICITY

Digoxin is commonly used in the treatment of chronic atrial fibrillation (AF) and heart failure. More than 10 per cent of patients receiving the drug have been found to have evidence of digoxin toxicity when admitted to hospital. Digoxin has a narrow therapeutic index (therapeutic concentration 1–2 ng/mL or 1.3–2.6 nmol/L) with toxicity occurring with serum concentrations >2.5 ng/mL. Serum concentration measurements must be taken at least 6 hours after the last dose. Toxicity can occur as a result of deliberate or accidental self-poisoning or more commonly from drug accumulation over a period of time, particularly in the elderly and patients with associated renal impairment. Drugs such as verapamil, captopril, quinine, quinidine, propafenone, flecainide, amiodarone, prazosin, spironolactone, tetracycline, erythromycin and carbenoxalone can also increase serum concentrations and predispose to toxicity. Agents causing hypokalaemia or intracellular potassium deficiency, hypomagnesaemia, hypercalcaemia and hypothyroidism can increase myocardial sensitivity to digoxin, despite satisfactory therapeutic concentrations.

Clinical presentation

Clinical features of toxicity include constitutional effects such as lethargy and weakness; gastrointestinal effects including anorexia, nausea and vomiting; neurological effects including confusion, weakness, paraesthesiae and, rarely, fits and acute psychosis; ocular disturbances including blurred vision, xanthopsia (yellow vision). Severe poisoning can cause hyperkalaemia (by inhibiting the myocardial membrane adenosine triphosphate (ATP) pump) and metabolic acidosis.

Digoxin toxicity can cause any arrhythmia, and various conduction disturbances. The commonest arrhythmia and, usually, an early sign of toxicity is the occurrence of ventricular ectopics, which frequently proceed to bigeminy, trigeminy or salvos.

Arrhythmias arise from several actions of the drug, which include:

- enhanced automaticity, which can give rise to various atrial and ventricular tachyarrhythmias;
- excess vagal stimulation, predisposing to sinus bradycardia and atrioventricular (AV) block;
- a direct depressive effect on nodal tissue, further contributing to bradyarrhythmias.

When these actions are present simultaneously, intoxication is highly likely and can cause the characteristic arrhythmia of atrial tachycardia with block. Other arrhythmias include junctional bradycardia, second or third degree AV block, ventricular tachycardia (VT) and ventricular fibrillation (VF). When concomitant medication elevates digoxin levels, the features of toxicity may depend on the agent added. For instance, quinidine predisposes to tachyarrhythmias, whereas verapamil and amiodarone predispose to bradycardia and AV block.

Management

If digoxin toxicity is suspected then the following steps should be taken:

- stop digoxin
- correct hypokalaemia if present
- check digoxin level
- monitor cardiac rhythm and correct any sustained haemodynamically significant arrhythmia that occurs.

For acute overdoses, oral activated charcoal should be given to absorb any cardiac glycoside remaining in the gut and to interrupt the enterohepatic circulation.

Ventricular ectopics, first degree AV block and AF with a slow rate but haemodynamic stability require no special therapy except drug withdrawal.

For haemodynamically unstable bradyarrhythmias and AV block IV atropine 0.3–1 mg every 3–5 minutes to a total of 0.04 mg/kg body weight should be given. If there is no response, then temporary transvenous pacing should be instituted. Beta-adrenergic agonists, such as isoprenaline, should be avoided because of the risk of precipitating more severe arrhythmias.

Supraventricular tachycardias can be treated with beta-blockers to control ventricular rate, but there is an increased risk of exacerbating AV conduction disturbances. Therefore, an ultra-short-acting beta-blocker, such as IV esmolol, should be used initially (see Appendix A). Ventricular tachyarrhythmias can be treated with lidocaine and magnesium. Magnesium possesses significant antiarrhythmic properties in the setting of digoxin toxicity. Phenytoin can be a useful treatment for ventricular or supraventricular tachycardias initiated by digoxin, and should be given as 50–100 mg IV as a slow bolus, every 5 minutes, to a dose not exceeding 600 mg.

For life-threatening arrhythmias, digoxin-specific antibodies (Digibind) are the treatment of choice. Digibind can be strikingly effective for life-threatening digoxin intoxication, especially when there are severe ventricular arrhythmias or hyperkalaemia. The reversal of toxicity is rapid with few adverse effects, apart from the development of hypokalaemia as the ATP pump activity is regained, and potassium is transferred from the extracellular to intracellular space. The use of Digibind should also be considered when more than 10 mg of digoxin has been ingested by previously healthy adults (4 mg in children), or when the steady-state serum concentration is greater than 10 ng/mL, or the serum potassium level is >5 mmol/L in the setting of severe intoxication. Digoxin levels may remain high, but most digoxin is bound to Fab fragments and is functionally inert. Therefore, measurement of digoxin levels is not reliable or useful following the administration of Digibind. Box 8.1 summarizes the calculation for the administration of Digibind.

The risk of provoking dangerous arrhythmias with electrical cardioversion is greatly increased in the presence of digoxin toxicity and is in proportion to the cardioversion energy used. Therefore, electrical cardioversion should only be used as a last resort for the treatment of life-threatening tachyarrhythmias, always starting at a low energy level (i.e. 10 J). Overdrive pacing can be considered in patients with refractory ventricular arrhythmias.

Haemodialysis is not useful because the drug has a large volume of distribution and is extensively tissue bound.

Box 8.1 Digibind indications and dosing regime

Digibind administration is indicated for:

Life-threatening arrhythmias or conduction disturbance
Serum potassium levels greater than 5 mmol/L in the presence of severe
   intoxication
Digoxin level >10 ng/mL

The dose of antibody depends on the body load of cardiac glycoside, which has to be counteracted. When requesting levels it is important to specify whether digoxin or digitoxin is to be measured as the assays differ.

To estimate the body load of digoxin or digitoxin from the amount ingested:

   The body load of digoxin or digitoxin = the amount
      ingested × 0.80 (mg)

To calculate the body load of digoxin or digitoxin from the plasma or serum digoxin or digitoxin concentration:

   The estimated body load (mg = plasma (serum) concentration of
      digoxin (ng/mL) × 0.0056 × body weight (kg)

The dose of antibody (Digibind) is about 60 times the body load (whether digoxin or digitoxin) rounded up to the nearest 40 mg. Sometimes up to 12 or 14 vials may be required.

TRICYCLIC ANTIDEPRESSANT OVERDOSE

Tricyclic antidepressants (TCADs) result in significant mortality when taken in overdose due to the cardiovascular effects of hypotension, myocardial depression and arrhythmias. The onset of toxicity is rapid with the majority of deaths occurring within a few hours of presentation.

Clinical presentation

Early clinical features are due to the anticholinergic effects of the drug, and include dilated pupils, dry skin, dry mouth, decreased bowel sounds (ileus), urinary retention and tachycardia. Cardiovascular toxicity can rapidly ensue with the development of hypotension, arrhythmias and asystole. Toxicity results primarily from effects on the myocardial cell action potential, direct effects on vascular tone and indirect effects mediated by the autonomic nervous system.

TCADs can inhibit the fast-acting sodium channel and are therefore similar to class 1A antiarrhythmic drugs. Consequently, TCADs can impair cardiac conduction and prolong repolarization. They also have a negative inotropic effect due to inhibition of calcium entry into myocytes. The inhibition of sodium channels is pH dependent with acidosis aggravating cardiotoxicity. Conversely, an increase in pH is protective by improving cardiac conduction and reducing negative inotropic effects. Impaired conduction in the His–Purkinje system slows propagation of the ventricular depolarization wave, and prolongs the QRS interval. QRS interval prolongation is the most distinctive feature of serious TCAD overdose, and is usually seen as a non-specific conduction delay on the electrocardiogram (ECG). A QRS duration >120 ms is a good predictor of cardiac and neurological toxicity, whereas a QRS duration >160 ms is predictive of ventricular arrhythmias. Prolongation of repolarization causes an increase in QT interval, predisposing to Torsade de Pointes. Non-uniform slowing may cause unidirectional block and re-entry circuits to develop, analogous to ischaemic myocardium, resulting in VT; VT may be difficult to distinguish from sinus tachycardia in the presence of prolonged QRS and PR intervals (P waves may be obscured by the preceding T wave). A 12-lead ECG may help reveal P waves not visible on a rhythm strip. VF is usually a terminal rhythm that occurs as a complication of VT or hypotension. The PR interval in TCAD overdose is often prolonged, but second or third degree AV block is rare. Sinus tachycardia is the most common rhythm disorder seen and is present in more than 50 per cent of patients.

Management

Management is generally supportive, with monitoring of respiration and cardiac rhythm. Owing to the possibility of rapid deterioration, intravenous access is recommended. A 12-lead ECG should be obtained because it may reveal QRS prolongation that is not evident on the single lead of a cardiac monitor.

The anticholinergic effects may delay gastric emptying, and a large, single dose of activated charcoal administration should be considered, particularly if ingestion has occurred within an hour of presentation.

Any hypoxia and electrolyte or metabolic disturbances should be corrected. Even in the absence of acidosis, if there is cardiac involvement (QRS prolongation >140 ms, ventricular arrhythmias) or hypotension, 50 mmol sodium bicarbonate should be administered slowly (see Appendix A). Because marked alkalosis can be physiologically detrimental, arterial blood pH should not exceed 7.5–7.55. Treatment for sinus tachycardia is not generally needed. First degree AV block requires no treatment, second (type II) or third degree AV block should be managed with temporary transvenous pacing. Any unstable ventricular tachyarrhythmias should be treated with direct current cardioversion (DCC); if recurrent, lidocaine should be administered. The use of other antiarrhythmic agents is limited, and may aggravate cardiotoxicity. Overdrive pacing should be considered in patients with refractory ventricular arrhythmias. Seizures should be treated with diazepam, as other anticonvulsant agents such as phenytoin may aggravate hypotension and arrhythmias. If seizures cannot be adequately controlled, paralysis and ventilation are indicated to prevent further acidosis. A fluid challenge often corrects mild hypotension and may facilitate the management of more severe hypotension, which can be treated with inotropic and vasopressor agents. Noradrenaline is the vasopressor of choice, although dobutamine may be effective in the presence of a low cardiac output but adequate filling pressures.

SUBSTANCE ABUSE

It is estimated that almost one in four people in developed countries have misused recreational drugs at some time during their life. Therefore, independent of clinical practice, most doctors will have to manage patients with the ill effects associated with recreational drug abuse at some point during their career. In addition to their effects on the central nervous system, many of these agents induce profound changes in the heart and circulation, which are responsible for a significant proportion of drug-related morbidity. The purpose of this section is to review the cardiovascular complications associated with some of the commonly misused recreational drugs.

Cocaine, crack, amphetamine and ecstasy

Pharmacology

These drugs all share similar adverse effects on the cardiovascular system, related predominantly to sympathetic nervous system activation. Cocaine and its freebase form, 'crack', act by inhibiting the noradrenaline re-uptake transporter in peripheral nerve terminals as well as stimulating central nervous system outflow. Circulating catecholamine concentrations can be elevated as much as five-fold in cocaine users. Cocaine has a short serum half-life of approximately 30–80 minutes, with 90 per cent being metabolized and excreted in the urine over a 2-week period. At high doses, cocaine can impair myocardial electrical conduction and contractility by blocking fast sodium and potassium channels and inhibiting calcium entry into myocytes. Amphetamine and its derivative ecstasy produce indirect sympathetic activation by releasing noradrenaline, dopamine and serotonin from central and autonomic nervous system terminals. The plasma half-life varies from as little as 5 hours to 20–30 hours depending on urine flow and pH (elimination is increased in acidic urine). Compared to cocaine, amphetamine lacks the local anaesthetic effect of inhibiting fast sodium channels.

Clinical effects
Sympathetic activation can lead to varying degrees of tachycardia, vasoconstriction, unpredictable blood pressure effects and arrhythmias, depending on the dose taken and the presence or absence of coexisting cardiovascular disease. Although hypertension is common, hypotension as a result of paradoxical central sympathetic suppression, a late relative catecholamine-depleted state or acute myocardial depression can occur. Myocardial depression may be caused by ischaemia, a direct toxic effect of the drug or mechanical complications (acute aortic rupture, tension pneumothorax, pneumopericardium, etc.).

Chest discomfort is a common symptom associated with cocaine, affecting 40 per cent of emergency department attenders following use of cocaine. Myocardial infarction occurs in up to 6 per cent of such patients in the United States, although a significant proportion may not offer a history of chest pain at all. Cocaine-related infarction usually occurs early (within 3 hours) after cocaine use, but events may occur several hours later owing to persistence of metabolites in the circulation. Both cocaine and amphetamine can cause myocardial ischaemia and infarction in patients with or without coronary artery disease. The underlying mechanisms are unclear, but may be related to the elevated catecholamine concentrations, which result in an increase in myocardial oxygen demand, coronary artery spasm, platelet aggregation and thrombus formation. Cocaine can produce a procoagulant effect by decreasing concentrations of protein C and antithrombin III, and potentiating thromboxane production. Chronic use of cocaine and amphetamine can cause repetitive episodes of coronary spasm and paroxysms of hypertension, which may result in endothelial damage, coronary artery dissection and acceleration of atherosclerosis. Creatine kinase concentrations can be elevated in both cocaine and amphetamine abusers, and are therefore not reliable indicators of myocardial injury. This elevation of creatine kinase is probably due to rhabdomyolysis. Consequently, serum troponin concentrations, which are more sensitive and specific for the detection of myocardial necrosis, should be measured in patients in whom cocaine- or amphetamine-related myocardial infarction (MI) is suspected.

Paroxysmal increases in blood pressure can lead to aortic dissection or valvular damage that increases the risk of endocarditis affecting mainly left-sided heart valves. Endocarditis is often associated with unusual organisms such as *Candida, Pseudomonas* or *Klebsiella*, and frequently has an aggressive clinical course with marked valvular destruction, abscess formation and a need for surgical intervention. Prolonged administration of cocaine or amphetamines can also lead to a dilated cardiomyopathy. Aetiological mechanisms include repeated episodes of subendocardial ischaemia and fibrosis, and myocyte necrosis produced by exposure to excessive catecholamine concentrations, infectious agents and heavy metal contaminants (manganese is present in some cocaine preparations). Non-cardiogenic pulmonary oedema and pulmonary hypertension can also occur with cocaine and amphetamine abuse. Although the precise underlying mechanism remains unknown, a direct toxic effect or alterations in central autonomic nervous system pulmonary vasculature regulation has been suggested.

The adverse cardiovascular changes and sympathetic stimulation associated with cocaine and amphetamine ingestion predispose to myocardial electrical instability, precipitating a wide and unpredictable range of supraventricular and ventricular tachyarrhythmias. The presence of fibrotic scars, myocardial ischaemia and left ventricular hypertrophy can act as a substrate for re-entrant arrhythmias. The class 1 antiarrhythmic effect of cocaine can impair cardiac conduction causing prolongation of the PR, QRS complex and QT intervals, and a wide range of bradyarrhythmias including sinus arrest and higher degrees of AV block.

Some cocaine users practise drug inhalation in association with a forced Valsalva manoeuvre (the positive ventilatory pressure increases drug absorption and therefore can enhance the drug's effect), which can, rarely, be complicated by a pneumothorax or pneumopericardium. Sudden cardiovascular collapse may occur as a result of myocardial ischaemia and infarction, arrhythmias, acute heart failure or mechanical complications.

Management

Similar principles apply to the management of the cardiovascular complications associated with these drugs. If the patient is agitated and anxious, then a benzodiazepine in sedative dosages should be administered as this can attenuate some of the cardiac and central nervous system toxicity.

In the treatment of hypertension, beta-blockers should be avoided, as they may be associated with unopposed alpha-mediated vasoconstriction leading to paradoxical increase in blood pressure and coronary artery vasoconstriction. The combined alpha- and beta-blocker drug, labetalol, is theoretically preferable to selective beta-blockers. However, the alpha-blocking effect is relatively weak and therefore labetalol can also exacerbate hypertension. Hypertension can be safely managed with either an alpha-blocker such as phentolamine or with vasodilators such as hydralazine, nitrates and nitroprusside. When hypertensive crises lead to the mechanical complication of aortic dissection or acute valve rupture, emergency cardiothoracic surgery may be required.

Myocardial ischaemia should be treated initially with oxygen, aspirin and benzodiazepine. If there is continuing ischaemia, then vasodilators such as nitrates or phentolamine should be administered in an attempt to reverse residual coronary artery spasm. Patients with persistent ST segment elevation should undergo primary angioplasty. Among patients undergoing coronary stenting, the potential of non-compliance with antiplatelet medication should be borne in mind when choosing the type of stent.

The majority of arrhythmias are short lived and terminate spontaneously as the drug is metabolized and cardiac function returns to normal. Consequently, antiarrhythmic agents should be avoided if possible. Supraventricular or ventricular tachyarrhythmias associated with haemodynamic compromise require urgent DCC. Sustained haemodynamically tolerated supraventricular arrhythmias should be treated initially with adenosine. In the presence of a hyperadrenergic state, the short-lived inhibitory effect of adenosine may be a disadvantage, allowing reinduction of the arrhythmia. If adenosine is unsuccessful or the arrhythmia rapidly returns, the co-administration of an alpha-blocker in combination with a beta-blocker may be effective. In 'body packers' suffering from overdose after rupture of ingested packets of cocaine, calcium antagonist may accelerate gastrointestinal drug absorption by inducing splanchnic vasodilatation. Furthermore, cocaine has a complex and highly variable effect on myocyte calcium metabolism, producing an unpredictable clinical response to calcium antagonist. For these reasons, it may be preferable to avoid giving calcium antagonists to patients suspected of cocaine abuse. Bradyarrhythmias can be treated with atropine; however, its effect may be attenuated in the presence of a hyperadrenergic state, and temporary cardiac pacing may be necessary. In the presence of sustained ventricular tachyarrhythmias, lidocaine and magnesium have an acceptable safety and efficacy profile (despite theoretical concerns relating to the shared class 1 effects of cocaine and lidocaine). There is currently no reliable information on the safety and efficacy of other antiarrhythmic drugs.

In animal studies using cocaine, the administration of sodium bicarbonate has been shown to have a beneficial effect on myocardial electrical stability. However, this may occur at the expense of inducing paradoxical intracellular acidosis or adverse systemic metabolic changes, leading to detrimental effects on myocardial function. Similarly, in severe cases of amphetamine overdose, a forced acid diuresis may be successful in rapidly clearing amphetamine from the blood and limiting toxicity, but major detrimental metabolic changes in the acid–base balance can be induced. These treatments require intensive and expert monitoring and should be performed only by clinicians with previous metabolic experience.

Lysergic acid diethylamide and psilocybin
Pharmacology
Lysergic acid diethylamide (LSD) and psilocybin (magic mushrooms) are commonly abused hallucinogenic agents that are structurally related, and have similar physiological, pharmacological and clinical effects. LSD is about 100 times more potent than psilocybin. Street mushrooms are often adulterated with LSD. Both drugs are indole derivatives and chemically resemble serotonin. Their mechanisms of action are complex and include agonist, partial agonist and antagonist effects at various serotonin receptors. The clinical effects are related to their serotonergic, dopaminergic and adrenergic activities. LSD is metabolized by the liver and has a plasma half-life of 100 minutes.

Clinical effects
The adrenergic effects of these drugs are usually mild and do not produce the profound sympathetic storms seen with cocaine and amphetamine. Symptoms corresponding to general sympathetic arousal include dilated pupils, tachycardia, hypertension and hyper-reflexia. Although

cardiovascular complications are rarely serious, supraventricular tachyarrhythmias and MI have been reported. Changes in serotonin-induced platelet aggregation and sympathetically induced arterial vasospasm have been suggested as mechanisms contributing to these complications.

Management

Management is usually supportive, as the majority of symptoms resolve within 12 hours. Agitated patients should be sedated with a benzodiazepine. The use of neuroleptic agents should be avoided as they can intensify toxic effects. Supraventricular arrhythmias can be treated with adenosine or verapamil. Apart from benzodiazepines, pharmacological intervention for mild to moderate hypertension is usually not required. Treatment for dangerously high blood pressure and myocardial ischaemia should follow the same general principles described for cocaine and amphetamine.

Narcotic analgesics

Pharmacology

Morphine and its semi-synthetic analogue heroin are the most commonly misused narcotic analgesics. When used alone or in combination with other drugs, they account for over 40 per cent of drug-related deaths. Heroin is slowly metabolized to morphine, which has a plasma half-life of 2–3 hours.

Clinical effects

Narcotic agents act centrally on the vasomotor centre to increase parasympathetic and reduce sympathetic activity. This effect, combined with histamine release from mast cell degranulation, can result in bradycardia and hypotension. Drug-induced bradycardia along with enhanced automaticity can precipitate an increase in atrial and ventricular ectopic activity, AF, idioventricular rhythm or potentially lethal ventricular tachyarrhythmias. Some narcotic drugs (such as the synthetic agent, dextropropoxyphene, a constituent of co-proxamol) have additional sodium channel blocking effects, causing ECG QRS prolongation, and further contributing to their pro-arrhythmic potential. It is recognized that methadone, commonly used in treating opioid addiction, delays cardiomyocyte repolarization, resulting in ECG QT prolongation, which is associated with Torsade de Pointes.

Bacterial endocarditis, affecting mainly right-sided cardiac structures, is a well-known complication of intravenous narcotic drug abuse, sometimes associated with pulmonary abscesses. Heroin overdose can cause non-cardiogenic pulmonary oedema, the onset of which can be delayed for up to 24 hours after admission. As the oedema fluid has the same protein concentration as plasma, and the pulmonary capillary wedge pressure is normal, a disruption in alveolar-capillary membrane integrity has been suggested as a mechanistic cause.

Management

Initial management centres around ensuring an adequate airway, breathing and circulation. In the presence of respiratory depression, severe hypotension and bradycardia, administration of repeated boluses or an infusion of a narcotic receptor antagonist, naloxone (Narcan), will be required, as detailed in Appendix A. In severe hypotension, the insertion of a pulmonary flow catheter may be needed to help guide fluid and inotropic administration, and avoid inappropriate administration of diuretics in patients with non-cardiogenic pulmonary oedema, which requires intensive ventilatory support.

There are no useful published data to guide selection of antiarrhythmic agents for the treatment of supraventricular and ventricular tachyarrhythmias. In the first instance, patients should be investigated, and hypoxic, metabolic and electrolyte deficits corrected. As the misused drug is rapidly metabolized, the majority of arrhythmias are short lived, and it is therefore preferable to avoid the use of antiarrhythmic agents where possible to minimize the risk of pro-arrhythmic interactions. If treatment is needed for supraventricular arrhythmia, conventional agents such as adenosine, beta-blockers, verapamil and digoxin have been recommended. Ventricular arrhythmias should be managed along conventional lines. Persistent bradycardia may require atropine or temporary cardiac pacing.

Volatile substance abuse

The abuse of volatile substances is an increasing problem amongst young male adolescents. The products used are legal, cheap and easily available. Abusers generally employ deep breathing techniques with the volatile substances contained in a plastic bag or bottle, a crisp packet or a soaked handkerchief to maximize the inhaled concentration of the substance.

Clinical effects

Following inhalation, feelings of euphoria, excitement and invulnerability can occur rapidly and are short lived. Cardiac arrhythmias are presumed to be the main cause of death from volatile substance abuse. Volatile substances may induce supraventricular or ventricular tachyarrhythmias by sympathetic activation or by myocardial sensitization to circulating catecholamines. Some abusers directly spray the substances into the oral cavity, which can result in intense vagal stimulation and a reflex bradycardia. Profound bradycardia can evolve into asystole or secondary ventricular tachyarrhythmias. Some volatile compounds can reduce sino-atrial node automaticity, prolong the PR interval and induce atrioventricular block. Myocardial ischaemia and infarction have been reported and are believed to be caused by a combination of coronary vasospasm, hypoxia or excessive sympathetic stimulation. Hypoxia can occur as a result of respiratory depression, aspiration, the placement of bags over the head and neck, intense laryngeal oedema and spasm, and the formation of carboxyhaemoglobin or methaemoglobin. Some volatile substances are structurally related to the agents used in general anaesthesia, and can therefore cause myocardial depression and hypotension. Chronic abuse can induce a poorly characterized cardiomyopathy.

Management

Patients should be managed in a calm non-threatening environment, with sedation if necessary. Hypoxia and chemical disturbances should be corrected to optimize myocardial electrical stability. Haemodynamically unstable tachyarrhythmias require prompt electrical cardioversion. Profound bradyarrhythmias may be treated cautiously with atropine or temporary cardiac pacing. Hypotension can be treated with intravenous fluids, guided by a pulmonary artery catheter, if necessary. Inotropic agents are best avoided, if possible, as they may induce refractory ventricular tachyarrhythmias in the electrically unstable myocardium. Calcium administration may help to reverse myocardial depression. In patients with sustained tachyarrhythmias, beta-blockers or amiodarone may help to combat sympathetic activation and are the antiarrhythmic drugs of choice. Cardiac ischaemia should be managed with oxygen, vasodilators and reperfusion treatment. Cardiomyopathies are treated conventionally.

Cannabis

Pharmacology

Cannabis is the most widely consumed recreational drug. It has a plasma half-life of 20–30 hours and can be detected in the urine for several days in occasional users, and up to months in heavy users.

Clinical effects

Cannabis has a biphasic effect on the autonomic nervous system, depending on the dose absorbed. Low or moderate doses can increase sympathetic and reduce parasympathetic activity, producing a tachycardia and an increase in cardiac output. In contrast, higher doses inhibit sympathetic and increase parasympathetic activity, resulting in bradycardia and hypotension. Reversible ECG abnormalities affecting the P and T waves, and the ST segment, have been reported. It is not clear whether these changes occur as a direct result of cannabis, independent of its effect on the heart rate.

Supraventricular and ventricular ectopic activity can occur, and arrhythmias possibly relating to cannabis use have been reported. In patients with ischaemic heart disease, cannabis increases the frequency of anginal symptoms at low levels of exercise and may be a trigger for the onset of an acute MI. This is believed to occur as a result of drug-induced increase in blood pressure, heart rate and myocardial contractility, increasing myocardial oxygen demand.

Management

In the absence of major underlying structural heart disease, the autonomically mediated changes in heart rate and blood pressure are usually well tolerated and therefore no treatment is needed. Where necessary, hypotension usually responds to intravenous fluid administration. For significant bradycardia, atropine can be administered. Patients presenting with unstable angina or MI should be treated conventionally.

KEY POINTS

- The abuse of recreational drugs is common and it is inevitable that doctors will have to manage and treat their associated ill effects.

- Recreational drugs are complex and can induce profound changes in cardiovascular function, both acutely and chronically.

- Recreational drugs are often taken together, which can result in complex synergistic interactions with potentially detrimental effects.

- A high index of suspicion with early intervention and management is often the key to successful treatment.

KEY REFERENCES

AHA Scientific Statement Management of Cocaine-Associated Chest Pain and Myocardial Infarction. *Circulation* 2008; **117**: 1897–1907.

Dick M, Curwin J, Tepper D. Digitalis intoxication recognition and management. *J Clin Pharmacol* 1991; **31**: 444–7.

Fisher BAC, Ghuran A, Vadamalai V, Antonios TF. Cardiovascular complications induced by cannabis smoking: a case report and review of the literature. *Emerg Med J* 2005; **22**: 679–80.

Ghuran A, Nolan J. Recreational drug abuse; issues for the cardiologist. *Heart* 2000; **83**: 627–33.

Kelly RA, Smith TW. Recognition and management of digitalis toxicity. *Am J Cardiol* 1992; **69**: 108G–19G.

Mittleman MA, Lewis RA, Maclure M, Sherwood JB, Muller JE. Triggering myocardial infarction by marijuana. *Circulation* 2001; **103**: 2805–9.

Osterwalder JJ. Patients intoxicated with heroin or heroin mixtures: how long should they be monitored? *Eur J Emerg Med* 1995; **2**: 97–101.

Toxbase (National Poisons Information Service): http://www.spib.axl.co.uk

Williams DR, Cole SJ. Ventricular fibrillation following butane gas inhalation. *Resuscitation* 1998; **37**: 43–5.

PERICARDITIS

BACKGROUND

Acute pericarditis is a clinical syndrome caused by inflammation of the pericardium and characterized by chest pain, a pericardial friction rub and electrocardiographic abnormalities. It is more common in adult males than in women and young children. Common causes include idiopathic, viral, bacterial, uraemia, post-myocardial infarction, trauma and neoplasms (Table 9.1). After myocardial infarction, pericarditis can occur within 1–4 days, or, less commonly, after 1–4 weeks as part of Dressler's syndrome, a systemic inflammatory condition thought to result from an autoimmune reaction to myocardial necrosis. The pericardial reaction can be purulent, haemorrhagic, fibrinous or serofibrinous. Complications may result in restriction of cardiac filling, either as a result of blood or fluid trapped in the pericardial sac (cardiac tamponade) or from thickening of the pericardium (constrictive pericarditis). These conditions may be prevented if diagnosis and management are undertaken early.

CLINICAL FEATURES

Pericarditis often presents with sharp chest pain, localized retrosternally or in the left precordial region, and exacerbated by breathing, coughing, moving or lying flat. The pain often radiates to the trapezius ridge, but may also radiate into the neck, jaw, arms, or upper abdomen and can therefore mimic an ACS or an acute abdomen. The pain is relieved by sitting up and leaning forward. As the pericardium is well innervated, acute inflammation may cause intense pain and initiate vagal reflexes. There may be a history of prodromal symptoms, which can include fever, malaise and myalgia. Dyspnoea may occur because of splinting of the chest from pain or because of significant accumulation of pericardial fluid (see Chapter 11).

Table 9.1 Causes of pericarditis

Infections	Viral: coxsackie B, echovirus, adenovirus, EBV, mumps, hepatitis B, HIV
	Bacterial: staphylococci, streptococci, rheumatic fever, *Haemophilus influenzae*, *Salmonella*, tuberculosis, *Neisseria meningitidis*, *Neisseria gonorrhoeae*, syphilis
	Fungal: histoplasmosis, *Candida*, aspergillosis
	Others: *Mycoplasma pneumoniae*, *Legionella*, psittacosis, rickettsiae, actinomycosis, amoebiasis, *Echinococcus*, *Nocardia*, toxoplasmosis
Neoplasms	Primary, e.g. mesothelioma, angiosarcoma, teratoma, fibroma
	Secondary, e.g. lung, breast, leukaemia, lymphoma, melanoma, Kaposi's sarcoma, colon
Connective tissue disease	SLE, Still's disease, rheumatoid arthritis, systemic sclerosis, mixed connective tissue disease, polyarteritis nodosa
Drug-induced	Hydralazine, methyldopa, minoxidil, procainamide, dantrolene, daunorubicin, doxorubicin, cyclophosphamide and methysergide
Post-myocardial injury	Post-MI, Dressler's syndrome, trauma, post-pericardiotomy, pacemaker insertion, cardiac diagnostic procedures
Other	Idiopathic, uraemia, hypothyroidism, sarcoidosis, Behçet disease, radiation, oesophageal rupture

A pericardial friction rub is often present and is best heard along the left sternal edge with the patient leaning forward. The persistence of the rub throughout inspiration and expiration as well as when the breath is held can help distinguish a pericardial rub from a left-sided pleural rub. Large effusions can compress the base of the left lobe of the lung, causing an area of dullness and bronchial breath sounds just below the angle of the left scapula (Ewart's sign).

DIAGNOSIS

General

Non-specific markers of inflammation including white cell count (WCC), erythrocyte sedimentation rate (ESR) and C-reactive protein (CRP) are usually raised. Cardiac enzymes may be elevated if the inflammation extends to the myocardium, and for this reason cardiac isoenzymes cannot always be used to differentiate between acute pericarditis and ACS. Cardiac troponins are frequently elevated, but do not necessarily indicate a worse outcome. Other specific haematological, biochemical and serological investigations are dependent on the suspected aetiology and include:

- urine and electrolytes (U&Es);
- antistreptolysin O titres, anti-Dnase B titre, throat swabs (acute rheumatic fever);
- blood cultures;
- acute and convalescent viral titres, monospot or Paul–Bunnell test (Epstein–Barr virus), cold agglutinins (mycoplasma), fungal precipitins;.
- sputum, urine and faecal samples for microbiology;
- Heaf test (tuberculosis);
- autoantibodies (lupus, rheumatoid arthritis, systemic sclerosis, etc.);
- thyroid function tests.

Chest x-ray can be normal, or the heart shadow may be enlarged, suggesting the presence of a pericardial effusion. There may be pleural effusions but pulmonary congestion, if present, indicates associated myocarditis.

Electrocardiogram

ECG changes (Figure 9.1) can occur a few hours or days after the onset of pericardial pain and are characterized initially by concordant, concave ST segment elevation in all leads except leads aVR, V1 and sometimes V2 (these leads show reciprocal ST depression). There is often PR segment depression associated with ST elevation (and sometimes PR elevation with ST depression). The following evolutionary changes then occur: isoelectric ST segment with flattened T waves, isoelectric ST segment with T inversion and finally reversion of T waves to normal. These changes are different from cardiac ischaemia (Table 9.2). It should be emphasized that they may not follow an exact sequence and some patients may present with only ST elevation and a return to normal without T inversion. Alternatively, T inversion may be the first sign, since the acute process was missed. Pericardial effusion can produce low voltage QRS complexes and electrical alternans (see Chapter 11).

Echocardiography

Echocardiography is valuable for determining the presence and size of a pericardial effusion and monitoring progress if the effusion is drained or treated conservatively. Furthermore, any contractile dysfunction resulting from myocarditis can also be detected.

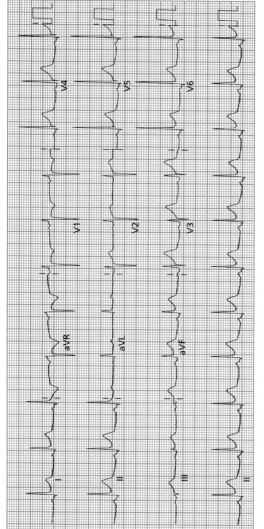

Figure 9.1 Electrocardiogram of a patient with an acute pericarditis.

Table 9.2 Progression of the electrocardiographic changes of pericarditis compared with myocardial infarction

Myocardial infarction	Pericarditis
Convex ST elevation	Concave ST elevation
ST elevation and T inversion	Isoelectric ST segment with T flattening and later T inversion
Loss of R-wave voltage and Q waves	Return to normal

MANAGEMENT

The first step is to establish whether the pericarditis is related to an underlying medical problem that requires specific therapy; for instance, uraemic pericarditis will require urgent dialysis.

Non-specific therapy consists of bed rest until pain and fever have disappeared, and the administration of anti-inflammatory agents such as aspirin (600–900 mg every 4–6 hours), ibuprofen (200–400 mg every 6 hours) or indomethacin (25–50 mg every 6 hours). In the randomized COPE study, the addition of colchicine to aspirin was shown to be more effective than aspirin monotherapy for the treatment of acute pericarditis. The dose given was 1-2 mg during the first 24 h, followed by a maintenance dose of 0.5-1 mg daily for 3 months. Combination therapy was associated with quicker symptom resolution as well as a much reduced recurrence rate. Similarly, the same combination was more effective than aspirin alone for recurrent episodes. With the exception of aspirin, anti-inflammatory drugs should be used cautiously in post-infarction pericarditis as they can affect scar formation and predispose to myocardial rupture. Some therapeutic studies have indicated that corticosteroid treatment is associated with more frequent recurrent pericarditis. In general, corticosteroids should be reserved for those with underlying rheumatalogic conditions or intolerance to the agents discussed above.

Antibiotics should be restricted to cases of purulent pericarditis and documented antibiotic-sensitive micro-organisms. Anticoagulants should be discontinued unless there is strong evidence for the development of thromboembolic complications. If anticoagulants must be continued, such as in patients with mechanical heart valves, intravenous heparin, which has a short half-life and whose action can easily be reversed with protamine sulphate, should be used. Patients should then be examined closely for the development of pericardial effusion.

Table 9.3 High-risk features of pericarditis

Large (≥ 2cm) circumferential pericardial effusion on echo
History of anticoagulant use
History of, or concurrent, malignancy (particularly lung, breast, leukaemia or lymphoma)
Chest trauma including surgery
Fever exceeding 38°C
Subacute onset (days to weeks)
Immunosuppression
Evidence for myocarditis
Atypical ECG evolution
Pulsus paradoxus
Significantly raised acute phase reactants and very high troponin

Adapted with permission from Spodick (2008) pp.: 398–9.

The diagnostic yield of pericardial aspiration is poor, and this procedure should not routinely be performed in acute pericardts. However, aspiration of the fluid may be needed to confirm a diagnosis, particularly if purulent disease is suspected, and/or to treat cardiac tamponade. Recurrent effusions may require the formation of a pericardial window, balloon pericardiotomy or the instillation of chemotherapeutic agents.

Acute idiopathic pericarditis is usually benign but may rapidly constrict or pursue a relapsing course before burning out. Late complications of pericarditis include pericardial fibrosis and/or calcification, resulting in constrictive pericarditis (particularly seen after episodes of tuberculous pericarditis), or a mixture of both effusive and constrictive pericardial disease. Studies have suggested that there are certain clinical and investigational features which may portend an adverse prognosis. A recent proposal suggested that cases of pericarditis without high-risk features (Table 9.3) can be observed for a few hours prior to discharge.

KEY POINTS

- There are a number of causes of acute pericarditis but idiopathic, viral and post-MI pericarditis are the commonest.

- Occasionally the pain of pericarditis can mimic an acute abdomen or MI; however, in the majority of cases pericarditis has characteristic clinical and electrocardiographic features.

- Most symptoms resolve with rest and non-steroidal anti-inflammatory agents.

- With the exception of aspirin, non-steroidal anti-inflammatory drugs and steroids should be used cautiously in post-infarction pericarditis as they can affect scar formation and predispose to myocardial rupture.

- Late complications include effusive and/or constrictive pericardial disease.

KEY REFERENCES

Imazio M, Bobbio M, Cecchi E, et al. Colchicine in addition to conventional therapy for acute pericarditis: results of the COlchicine for acute PEricarditis (COPE) trial. *Circulation* 2005; **112**: 2012–16.

Ivens EL, Munt BI, Moss RR. Pericardial disease: what the general cardiologist needs to know. *Heart* 2007; **93**: 993–1000.

Maisch B. Pericardial disease, with a focus on etiology, pathogenesis, pathophysiology, new diagnostic imaging methods, and treatment. *Curr Opin Cardiol* 1994; **9**: 379–88.

Oakley CM. Myocarditis, pericarditis and other pericardial disease. *Heart* 2000; **84**: 449–54.

Spodick DH. Risk prediction in pericarditis: who to keep in hospital. *Heart* 2008; **94**: 398–9.

CARDIAC TRAUMA

BACKGROUND

In developed countries, cardiac trauma represents one of the leading causes of death in those under the age of 40 years. Young males are more likely to be affected than females. Road traffic accidents and physical violence are responsible for the majority of cases, although the incidence of iatrogenic causes as a result of intravascular and intracardiac catheterization as well as cardiopulmonary resuscitation (CPR) is currently rising. Advances in initial resuscitation and surgical management mean more patients are surviving the initial insult.

Cardiac trauma is divided into penetrating and non-penetrating injuries. Both mechanisms can lead to myocardial rupture, contusion, laceration, pericardial insult, coronary injury, valvular damage, arrhythmias and conduction abnormalities. Cardiac trauma is easily overlooked as attention is diverted to more obvious skeletal and multisystem injuries. As a result, haemodynamic instability can rapidly develop with devastating results. A high index of clinical suspicion with the early use of diagnostic techniques is essential and is often the key to successful management. It is important for physicians to have a good working knowledge of cardiac trauma to enable them to diagnose the occurrence of these conditions and manage the non-surgical components.

NON-PENETRATING CARDIAC TRAUMA

Non-penetrating cardiac trauma usually occurs following the application of direct external physical forces to the chest wall. The incidence of cardiac damage following this type of injury is estimated to be 10–16 per cent. Non-penetrating cardiac trauma most often is the result of road traffic

Box 10.1 Consequences of non-penetrating cardiac trauma

Myocardium
- Contusion
- Laceration
- Rupture
  - Free wall
  - Septum
  - Valvular apparatus

Conduction disturbances
- Aneurysm, pseudoaneurysm

Pericardial injury
- Laceration
- Pericarditis
- Post-pericardiotomy syndrome
- Constrictive pericarditis

Aortic dissection

Coronary artery injury
- Laceration
- Dissection
- Fistulae
- Rupture
- Thrombosis

- Bundle branch block

- Bifascicular block
- Atrioventricular block
- Atrial arrhythmias
- Ventricular tachyarrhythmias
- Sinus node dysfunction

Commotio cordis (sudden cardiac death)

accidents (as the heart is compressed between the steering wheel or seat belt, and the sternum and spine) but can also occur as the result of falls, fights and sporting injuries. Box 10.1 summarizes the injuries that can develop as a consequence of non-penetrating cardiac trauma.

Cardiac contusion is considered the most common injury to the heart following blunt trauma. Cardiac contusion usually produces no significant symptoms and can easily go unrecognized. Subepicardial and subendocardial petechiae, bruising, haematoma, lacerations and full-thickness myocardial damage, later followed by necrosis, fibrosis and aneurysm formation, can occur. The key symptom is precordial pain resembling that of myocardial infarction (MI) but unrelieved with nitrates. Other sites of chest trauma may confuse the clinical picture, but unlike injury to the thoracic wall, pain from cardiac contusion is not affected by breathing. There may be inappropriate tachycardia, gallop rhythm and a pericardial rub. The electrocardiogram (ECG) may show non-specific ST-T wave changes (Figure 10.1), findings of pericarditis, loss of R-wave amplitude and even pathological Q waves depending on the degree of injury. Localized injury to the conducting system can give rise to varying degrees of atrioventricular (AV) block, intraventricular conduction defects or bundle branch block. Supraventricular tachycardias, atrial fibrillation

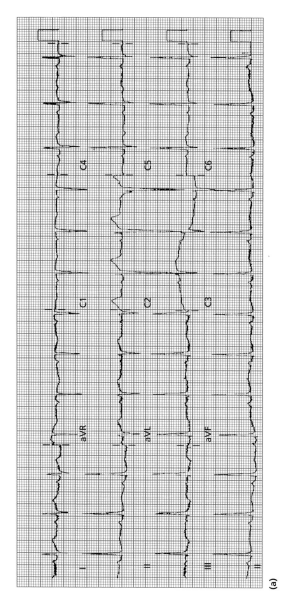

(a)

Figure 10.1(a) Non-penetrating cardiac injury sustained during a motor vehicular accident. Note the non-specific ST-T wave changes. There is T-wave inversion in lead III, and flattening in II and aVF. There was notching of the T wave in leads V3–V6. Reprinted with permission from Moriaty A. (1999) p. 578.

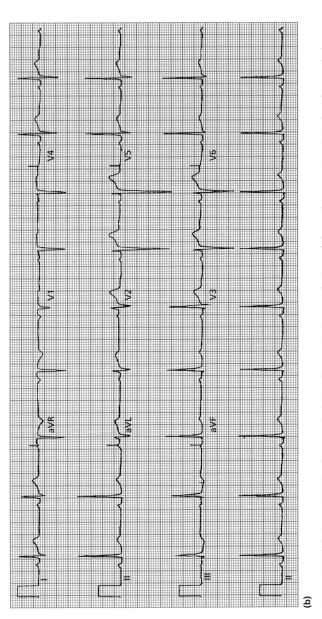

(b)

Figure 10.1(b) Repeat ECG a few weeks later demonstrates resolution of these changes. Reprinted with permission from Moriaty A. (1999) p. 578.

(AF), atrial and ventricular ectopics, ventricular tachycardia (VT) and ventricular fibrillation (VF) can also occur.

Cardiac-specific enzymes such as CK-MB isoenzyme, troponin T or troponin I can be used to make a diagnosis of cardiac contusion. Transthoracic echocardiography may show pericardial effusion, regional wall motion abnormalities, valve dysfunction and chamber enlargement. Up to 25 per cent of trauma patients cannot be satisfactorily imaged with transthoracic echocardiography and a transoesophageal echocardiogram (TOE) is a superior alternative. With the exception of anticoagulation and thrombolytic therapy, the treatment of cardiac contusion is similar to that of acute coronary syndrome (ACS). Arrhythmia or cardiogenic shock can occur within the first 48 hours after presentation. Therefore cardiac monitoring is essential in the initial phase if there is echocardiographic or marked ECG change. Troponin is released earlier than in classical ACS; therefore, when negative on admission, troponin should be rechecked 4–6 hours later. In uncomplicated cases treatment is initially with bed rest and analgesia. Non-steroidal anti-inflammatory drugs are not advised as they can interfere with myocardial healing. Complete recovery usually occurs, as patients are often young with an otherwise healthy heart. Some patients may develop left ventricular impairment as healing is by fibrosis in a similar manner as following ACS.

CARDIAC RUPTURE

Rupture of the free wall, interventricular septum, heart valves, papillary muscles or chordae tendineae can occur acutely owing to the direct force of the injury or may be delayed up to 2 weeks resulting from necrosis. Rupture of the thoracic aorta commonly occurs at the aortic isthmus, just below the origin of the left subclavian artery. These complications are usually fatal. Patients may present with signs and symptoms of acute cardiac tamponade, severe congestive heart failure with a new murmur or haemorrhagic shock. If indicated, pericardiocentesis may be life saving. Meticulous fluid resuscitation and early surgical intervention is the definitive treatment for most patients.

PERICARDIAL INJURY

Trauma to the pericardium can range from contusion to laceration or rupture allowing herniation of the heart. Clinical findings include a pericardial friction rub and ST-T wave changes on the ECG characteristic of pericarditis. Complications such as haemopericardium and tamponade can occur. In the case of cardiac herniation, the heart becomes entrapped, there may be impaired filling and occasionally compression of the coronary arteries. There may be evidence of a displaced heart and pneumopericardium on a chest x-ray. The ECG can show a new shift in axis or bundle branch block. The only therapy for cardiac herniation is surgical repositioning. Uncomplicated pericarditis can be treated with non-steroidal anti-inflammatory agents. Recurrent pericardial effusions associated with pericardial pain, pyrexia and a friction rub can sometimes occur. It is similar to the post-pericardiotomy syndrome and is treated with non-steroidal anti-inflammatory agents. Constrictive pericarditis can occur as a late sequel and the treatment is total pericardiectomy.

CORONARY ARTERY INJURY

Coronary artery trauma can lead to laceration, dissection, rupture and fistulae formation. ACS can occur if a coronary artery becomes occluded. A previously normal coronary artery may sustain disruption of the intima, subintimal haemorrhage and obstructive intraluminal thrombus formation on the injured arterial wall. The left anterior descending artery is most frequently affected due to its anterior position, followed by the proximal right coronary artery. The circumflex and left main stem are rarely affected. It may be impossible to differentiate from cardiac contusion without the use of coronary angiography. In patients with continuing pain and ECG changes consistent with evolving ACS it is reasonable to undertake coronary angiography with a view to percutaneous coronary intervention (PCI). However, this must be balanced against the risks in a patient with multiple associated injuries as antiplatelets and anticoagulation are required. Discussion with senior colleagues is essential.

COMMOTIO CORDIS

Sudden death may occur in young sport participants when a small hard ball (such as a cricket ball) or other projectile (lacrosse ball, hockey puck, karate kick) strikes the victim in the precordium. This phenomenon is termed commotio cordis and affects children and adolescents 5–15 years of age without pre-existing heart disease. It is the second most common cause of sudden cardiac death in young athletes after hypertrophic cardiomyopathy. Characteristically, there is no structural damage to the thoracic cavity or heart. The causative precordial blows are often not perceived as unusual for the sporting event involved or of sufficient magnitude to cause death. It is believed that an appropriately timed precordial blow, during the electrically vulnerable phase of ventricular repolarization (15–30 ms before the T-wave peak), can induce a ventricular tachyarrhythmia and subsequently death. At present, early basic and advanced life support, and ensuring adequate chest protection, are the only effective treatments against this phenomenon.

PENETRATING CARDIAC TRAUMA

Penetrating cardiac trauma is increasingly common with the majority being caused by gunshot and stab wounds, although shrapnel, fractured ribs, intracardiac diagnostic and therapeutic catheters can also produce penetrating cardiac injury. Penetrating wounds often result in laceration of the pericardium, as well as the underlying myocardium. One or more chambers, the interventricular and interatrial septa, valvular apparatus and coronary arteries may be involved. Box 10.2 summarizes the complications of penetrating cardiac trauma. In the case of stab wounds, the chamber most commonly involved is the right ventricle because of its anterior position followed by the left ventricle. Forty per cent of penetrating cardiac injuries are to the ventricles. Twenty-three per cent are to the right atrium and 3 per cent to the left atrium. Clinical presentation is dependent on the size of the wound and the location of the structures injured. If the pericardium remains open, blood can pass freely

---

Box 10.2 Consequences of penetrating cardiac trauma

Myocardium
- Laceration
  - Free wall
  - Septum
  - Valvular apparatus
  - Coronary arteries

Pericardial injury
- Haemopericardium
- Pneumopericardium
- Pericarditis
- Post-pericardiotomy syndrome

Conduction disturbances
- Bundle branch block
- Bifascicular block
- Atrioventricular block
- Atrial arrhythmias
- Ventricular tachyarrhythmias

into the mediastinum and pleural space, causing haemorrhagic shock and massive haemothorax on chest x-ray. This is commonly seen in large or right ventricular wounds. However, if the pericardium does not permit free drainage because its opening has been obstructed by a blood clot, adjacent lung tissue or other structures, then blood accumulates within the pericardial space, causing cardiac tamponade. Under these circumstances, the chest x-ray will show a normal size cardiac silhouette, as the acute and rapid accumulation of fluid within the pericardial space does not allow distension of the pericardium. Echocardiography can be useful for diagnosing pericardial effusions, foreign bodies in the heart and intracardiac shunts.

Initial management includes securing the airway, establishing venous access and appropriately administered intravenous fluids and blood. The offending object should remain *in situ* until exploratory surgery can be carried out. Patients who fail to respond to resuscitation and suddenly decompensate, should undergo immediate thoracotomy and repair of any treatable cardiac trauma. The incidence of late sequelae can be as high as 20 per cent and includes atrial and ventricular septal defects, tricuspid and mitral valve lacerations, and coronary injury. These complications may be missed on initial examination, only becoming apparent after a few days or weeks because of fibrous retraction of wound edges, resolution of oedema, ventricular enlargement and lysis of occluding clots. It is therefore essential that all post-cardiac trauma patients are closely monitored while in hospital and also in the outpatient clinic. Not surprisingly, penetrating cardiac injuries are usually immediately fatal, with the victim dying before reaching hospital.

KEY POINTS

- Cardiac trauma is a leading cause of death under the age of 40 years.

- It is divided into penetrating and non-penetrating injuries, which can both lead to myocardial rupture, contusion, laceration, pericardial insult, coronary injury, valvular damage, arrhythmias and conduction abnormalities.

- It is easily overlooked and should always be considered in anyone presenting with skeletal and multisystem injuries.

- A high index of clinical suspicion with the early use of diagnostic techniques is essential and is often the key to successful management.

KEY REFERENCES

Anderson DR. The diagnosis and management of non-penetrating cardiothoracic trauma. *Br J Clin Pract* 1993; **47**: 97–103.

Bansal, MK et al. Myocardial contusion injury: redefining the diagnostic algorithm. *Emerg Med J* 2005; **22**: 465–9.

Jackson L, Stewart A. Use of troponin for the diagnosis of myocardial contusion after blunt chest trauma. *Emerg Med J* 2005; **22**: 193–5.

Moriaty A. Myocardial contusion caused by seat belt. *Br J Cardiol* 1999; **6**: 577–9.

Westaby S, Odell JA. *Cardiothoracic Trauma*. London: Arnold, 1999.

CARDIAC TAMPONADE

BACKGROUND

Cardiac tamponade is an emergency clinical syndrome that occurs when blood or fluid fills the pericardial space, raising intrapericardial pressure and preventing ventricular diastolic filling. Consequently, venous pressures are greatly increased, and there is a reduction in stroke volume and cardiac output with the development of shock. The development of tamponade relates to the rapidity of fluid accumulation and the distensibility of the pericardium rather than the quantity of fluid. If accumulation is rapid, or if left ventricular function is compromised for other reasons, as little as 250 mL may be sufficient to produce tamponade. In contrast, it may take in excess of a litre of fluid to produce tamponade if it accumulates over a long period of time. Some common causes of cardiac tamponade are listed in Box 11.1.

CLINICAL PRESENTATION

Patients typically present with cardiogenic shock, with hypotension, cold-clammy peripheries, oligo-anuria and associated agitation. Untreated, this condition can be rapidly fatal. In the setting of a more slowly developing tamponade, patients appear less ill and may present with anorexia, weakness and signs of biventricular failure such as shortness of breath, peripheral oedema and hepatomegaly. There may be an accompanying tachycardia, and the presence of pulsus paradoxus (an inspiratory decrease in amplitude of the palpated pulse or measured blood pressure) is supportive of the diagnosis. The jugular venous pressure (JVP) is markedly elevated with a prominent x descent and absent y descent. A positive Kussmaul's sign (an inspiratory increase in the JVP) is rare in cardiac tamponade. Its presence suggests that an organizing

Box 11.1 Causes of cardiac tamponade

- Malignant disease
- Post-infective pericarditis
- Rupture of the free wall post-myocardial infarction
- Uraemia
- Iatrogenic; post-diagnostic (cardiac catheterization) or therapeutic procedures (pacemaker electrode insertion, angioplasty, etc.), anticoagulation
- Chest trauma
- Radiation
- Hypothyroidism
- Dissecting aortic aneurysm
- Post-pericardiotomy syndrome
- Dressler's syndrome
- Connective tissue diseases, e.g. rheumatoid arthritis, systemic lupus erythematosus, etc.
- Idiopathic

process and epicardial constriction is present, in addition to an effusion. The apex beat may not be palpable and the heart sounds are soft or even absent. There may be a pericardial friction rub.

In addition to a sinus tachycardia, the electrocardiogram (ECG) may show abnormalities of pericarditis, low voltage complexes and electrical alternans (alteration in QRS amplitude on a beat-to-beat basis as the heart continually alters its axis within the fluid-filled pericardial sac). The chest x-ray can show an enlarged globular heart shadow if the effusion is chronic or a normal cardiac silhouette if the tamponade develops acutely as seen during cardiac rupture or laceration. The lung fields are usually clear.

Although cardiac tamponade is very much a clinical diagnosis, echocardiography is the definitive investigation. Echocardiography will show the effusion and demonstrate the best approach for drainage. In tamponade, diastolic collapse of the low-pressure right heart chambers is evident, with right ventricular collapse being a more specific finding than right atrial collapse. Doppler indices showing reduced mitral and increased tricuspid inflow velocities with respiration are also specific features for demonstrating tamponade. Echocardiography can also exclude other causes of systemic venous hypertension and arterial hypotension such as constrictive pericarditis, cardiac dysfunction and right ventricular dysfunction.

MANAGEMENT

If haemodynamic compromise is present, intravenous fluids or inotropic agents can be administered to maintain haemodynamic support, while preparing the patients for pericardiocentesis (see below). Cardiac tamponade associated with cardiac trauma or aortic dissection requires immediate surgical intervention.

Pericardiocentesis

- Pericardial aspiration should ideally be performed with full x-ray screening, rhythm monitoring and resuscitation facilities readily available. Echocardiography can be used to guide pericardial aspiration as it allows visualization of the pericardial space, the myocardium and the aspiration needle. It can therefore give an indication of the best line of approach.

- The patient is placed at 30–45° to pool the pericardial fluid anteriorly and inferiorly. The patient is then connected to an ECG monitor.

- A long 18-gauge needle should be used. The V1 lead from an ECG machine can be connected to the metal hub of the needle via a sterile alligator clip to provide continuous monitoring from the tip of the puncture needle.

- Although several sites have been advocated for pericardiocentesis, the subxiphoid approach is preferred as it is extrapleural and avoids the coronary, pericardial and internal mammary arteries. The skin is cleaned and lignocaine infiltrated between the left side of the xiphisternum and the adjacent left costal margin, with the point directed towards the left shoulder, 45° to the skin.

- The needle is advanced while periodically aspirating and injecting small amounts of lignocaine. The needle is advanced until fluid is aspirated, indicating that the needle has reached the pericardial space. If using ECG monitoring, ST elevation indicates that the tip of the needle is in contact with the myocardium. Alternatively, the injection of a few millilitres of contrast media can be used to determine if the needle is in the pericardial space or within a cardiac chamber. If the contrast media swirls and is rapidly dispersed, then the needle is in a cardiac chamber. By contrast, the sluggish layering of contrast media inferiorly indicates that the needle is within the pericardial space. When using echocardiography rather than x-ray screening, injection of a few millilitres of agitated saline can be used to confirm the tip position by observing the appearance of microbubbles within the pericardial space. Failure of the bloody fluid to clot is further evidence that it is not from within the heart.

- The syringe is removed and a guidewire inserted under radiological or echocardiographic control. A pre-dilated pigtail drainage catheter is then inserted. Fluid can then be aspirated from the catheter. Removal of only 100 mL can produce a dramatic improvement in haemodynamic status. A connection is made to a collection bag if there is any possibility of fluid re-accumulating.

- Pericardial fluid should be sent for microbiology (microscopy, aerobic and anaerobic culture and sensitivity, including requests for fungal and tuberculous investigations), biochemistry (protein and glucose) and cytology.

- The catheter is generally removed after 24–48 hours, to reduce the chance of infection.

- A post-procedure chest x-ray is obtained to exclude a pneumothorax.

Rarely, following the removal of large amounts of pericardial fluid, sudden ventricular dilatation and acute pulmonary oedema may develop. This is probably related to a sudden increase in pulmonary venous blood flow, following the relief of pericardial compression in the presence of ventricular dysfunction.

KEY POINTS

- Cardiac tamponade is a clinical diagnosis caused by a critically increased volume of fluid within the pericardium obstructing inflow of blood to the ventricles.

- Consider the diagnosis in any patient in a haemodynamically collapsed state, with a raised JVP, reduced heart sounds, low-voltage complexes on the ECG and clear lung fields.

- Pericardiocentesis should be done only by those experienced in performing the procedure.

KEY REFERENCES

Callahan JA, Seward JB, Nishimura RA, et al. Two dimensional echocardiographically guided pericardiocentesis: experience in 117 consecutive patients. *Am J Cardiol* 1985; **55**: 476–84.

Guberman B, Fowler NO, Engel PJ, Gueron M, Allen JM. Cardiac tamponde in medical patients. *Circulation* 1981; **64**: 633–40.

Krikorian JG, Hancock EW. Pericardiocentesis. *Am J Med* 1978: **65**: 808–14.

APPENDICES

APPENDIX A: INTRAVENOUS CARDIAC DRUG REGIMENS

Drug	Indication	Side effects	Pharmacokinetics	Dosing regimen	Comments/Cautions/Contraindications
Abciximab	During PCI for ACS	Major and minor bleeding. Thrombocytopenia	Half-life = 10 min but effect on platelets up to 48 hours	IV or intracoronary bolus 250 µg/kg followed by infusion of 0.125 µg/kg/h for 12 hours	Thrombocytopenia occurs in 0.4–1% of patients and improves within 5–10 days. Readministration within 30 days is associated with a higher risk of thrombocytopenia (4%)
Adenosine	Narrow complex tachycardia (SVT)	Flushing, chest pain, headache, dyspnoea, bronchospasm, nausea, excess sinus or AV node inhibition (bradycardia)	Half-life = 10–30 s. Rapidly metabolized by erythrocytes and endothelial cells	Initially 6 mg through a large central or peripheral vein followed by a flush of 10 mL saline. If necessary a further 3 doses each of 12 mg can be administered every 1–2 min	Dipyridamole potentiates the effect of adenosine. Methylxanthines (theophylline, caffeine) competitively antagonize the adenosine receptors and therefore higher doses may be needed. Contraindications: asthmatics, second or third degree AV block and sick sinus syndrome

| Adrenaline (epinephrine) | Cardiac arrest Anaphylaxis Inotropic support | Tachycardia, arrhythmias, hypertension, hypokalaemia, hyperglycaemia, headache, anxiety, tremor, sweating | Half-life = 2 min β_1- and β_2-receptor agonist, high-dose α-adrenergic vasoconstrictive effect | Cardiac arrest: IV = 1 mg (10 mL of 1:10000 or 1 mL of 1:1000). Repeat as per resuscitation guidelines Anaphylaxis: initially, IM = 0.5 mg (0.5 mL of 1:1000). Repeat after 5 min in the absence of clinical improvement. In some cases several doses may be needed. In severely ill patients with circulatory collapse, give IV 500 μg (5 mL of 1 in 10000) at a rate of 100 μg/min with ECG monitoring. Also give chlorpheniramine 10–20 mg IM/IV and hydrocortisone 100–500 mg IM/IV Inotropic support: 5 mL of 1:1000 in 45 mL of 5% dextrose or normal saline (this gives a concentration of 100 μg/ mL). The usual infusion dose ranges between 0.01 and 0.5 μg/kg/min. Higher infusion doses are acceptable depending on the clinical condition | Cautions: ischaemic heart disease, diabetes mellitus, hyperthyroidism and hypertension |

Appendix A: (*Contd*)

Drug	Indication	Side effects	Pharmacokinetics	Dosing regimen	Comments/Cautions/Contraindications
Alteplase (Actilyse, rt-PA)	STEMI Pulmonary embolism (PE)	Minor and major haemorrhages, rash, nausea and vomiting	Half-life = 4 min. Metabolized by the liver. Binds to fibrin-associated plasminogen to form plasmin, which in turn breaks down fibrinogen and fibrin	MI: given as an accelerated regimen: IV 15 mg bolus, followed by 0.75 mg/kg (maximum 35 mg) over 30 min, then 0.5 mg/kg (maximum 35 mg) over 60 min. Give heparin IV 5000 U before commencing rt-PA, followed by 1000 U/h after completion of the rt-Pa infusion. Aim for an aPTT 50–75 s (1.5–2.5 times control) PE: IV 10 mg over 1–2 min, followed by 90 mg over 2 h. Maximum 1.5 mg/kg in patients <65 kg. Give heparin as mentioned above	At present, few absolute contraindications as many are now relative, which needs interpreting within the clinical context. See section on thrombolysis, in Chapter 1
Amiodarone	Accessory pathway tachycardias, atrial fibrillation, atrial flutter Ventricular tachyarrhythmias Cardiac arrest (VF)	Pulmonary fibrosis, hyper/hypothyroidism, corneal microdeposits, skin photosensitivity and discolouration, pro-arrhythmic effect recorded though rare	Half-life = 25–110 days. Hepatic metabolism, lipid soluble with extensive distribution in the body	During cardiac arrest: VF/pulseless VT: amiodarone 300 mg, made up to 20 mL with 5% dextrose (can be given peripherally). A further dose of 150 mg may be given for recurrent or refractory VF/VT, followed by an infusion of 1 mg/min	Can increase digoxin and warfarin levels. Contraindications: sinus or AV node disease (unless fitted with a pacemaker) iodine sensitivity, pregnancy, breast feeding, thyroid dysfunction (relative)

	Indications	Side effects	Pharmacokinetics	Dose	Notes
				for 6h and then 0.5mg/min to a maximum daily dose of 2g. Stable tachyarrhythmias: 150mg diluted in 5% dextrose to a volume of 20mL given over 10min; this can be followed by a further dose of 150mg if needed. Alternatively, a dose of 300mg in 100mL 5% dextrose over 1h can be given. Follow with a continuous infusion of 900mg in 5% dextrose over 24h. Maximum recommended dose is 1.2g in 24h (European data sheet recommendation) although current resuscitation guidelines advocate that up to 2g in 24h can be used	Administration via a central line is preferable to avoid thrombophlebitis during prolonged infusions. However, a large peripheral line is acceptable in the short term until arrangements can be made to place a central line by skilled personnel
Atenolol	Acute management of supraventricular tachyarrhythmias (including atrial fibrillation and atrial flutter) ACS Angina Hypertension	Hypotension, bronchospasm, negative inotrope and chronotrope, peripheral ischaemia	Half-life = 6–9h. Excreted by the kidney, cardioselective, not lipid soluble	IV 2.5–10mg at a rate of 1mg/min	Acts synergistically with digoxin to control atrial fibrillation. Contraindications: heart rate less than 60 bpm, PR interval >0.24s, second or third degree AV block, systolic arterial pressure <100mmHg.

Appendix A: (*Contd*)

Drug	Indication	Side effects	Pharmacokinetics	Dosing regimen	Comments/Cautions/Contraindications
					uncontrolled heart failure (once stabilized an oral beta-blocker can be cautiously given), severe chronic obstructive pulmonary disease, history of asthma, severe peripheral vascular disease, Prinzmetal's angina, cocaine and amphetamine toxicity, and phaeochromocytoma
Atropine sulphate	Bradyarrhythmias Cardiac arrest (asystole)	Tachycardia, dry mouth, blurred vision (difficulties with visual accommodation), urinary retention, constipation	Rapidly cleared from the blood and is distributed throughout the body. Incompletely metabolized in the liver and excreted in the urine as unchanged drug and metabolite. A half-life of about 4 h has been reported	IV 0.3–1 mg every 3–5 min to a total of 3 mg or 0.04 mg/kg body weight. During resuscitation IV 3 mg bolus (see resuscitation guidelines)	Contraindications: angle closure glaucoma (pupillary dilation can increase intraocular pressure), myasthenia gravis, prostatic enlargement (can precipitate urinary retention). These effects, however, are not relevant to either the cardiac arrest situation or immediate post-resuscitation care

Bivalirudin	Anticoagulation during PCI and treatment of ACS	Major and minor bleeding	Half-life = 25 min. Rapid onset of action with peak concentrations 15 min after IV bolus. Eliminated mainly by renal excretion	For PCI: IV bolus of 0.75 mg/kg followed by infusion of 1.75 mg/kg/h. In medical treatment of ACS: IV bolus of 0.1 mg/kg followed by infusion of 0.25 mg/kg/h for up to 72 hours	Caution in renal failure Monitor ACT
Calcium chloride 10% or calcium gluconate 10%	Hyperkalaemia Hypocalcaemia EMD arrest Calcium antagonist toxicity	Bradycardias and arrhythmias	Transient effects	IV 10 mL of the 10% solution. Give slowly	Avoid adding to solutions containing bicarbonate, phosphates or sulphates. Use separate IV access
Digoxin	Rate control atrial fibrillation, atrial flutter Heart failure	Anorexia, nausea, confusion, vomiting, visual disturbance. Arrhythmias including ventricular ectopy and bigeminy, paroxysmal atrial tachycardia with block, heart block, idioventricular rhythm, ventricular tachycardia	Half-life = 36 h. Excreted mainly by the kidney. Peak effect may take up to 2 h. Therapeutic concentration 1–2 ng/mL (1.3–2.6 nmol/L). Toxic range >2.5 ng/mL	For atrial fibrillation, give 250–500 µg (orally) every 8 h for 24 h, then 125–250 µg daily thereafter. A loading dose is not necessarily required for use in mild heart failure. In renal impairment, reduce dose. For urgent loading, give IV 0.5–1 mg (diluted in 50 mL of 5% dextrose or normal saline) over at least 2 h	Reduce dose in elderly and in renal failure. Hypokalaemia, hypomagnesaemia, hypercalcaemia, and hypothyroidism increase myocardial sensitivity to digoxin. Cautious administration in patients with hypertrophic obstructive cardiomyopathy and atrial fibrillation. Contraindications: patients with Wolff–Parkinson–White syndrome, second or third degree AV block

Appendix A: (*Contd*)

Drug	Indication	Side effects	Pharmacokinetics	Dosing regimen	Comments/Cautions/Contraindications
Dobutamine	Inotropic support in cardiogenic shock	Tachycardias, arrhythmias, hypertension hypokalaemia	Half-life = 2.4 min. β_1-adrenergic receptor agonist, lesser β_2- and α-agonist effects	Given as an IV infusion between 2.5 and 20 µg/kg/min. Can be given peripherally. See Table A.1 for infusion rates according to body weight	Central haemodynamic monitoring recommended. Infusion can be given via a peripheral line
Dopamine	Low doses for renal perfusion Moderate doses for cardiac inotropic support High dose for peripheral vasoconstriction	As for dobutamine	Half-life = 5 min. Low doses stimulate renal dopamine receptors, therefore improving renal blood flow. Moderate doses stimulate β_1-receptors. High doses stimulate α-receptors	2.5 µg/kg/min for renal perfusion. 5–20 µg/kg/min for inotropic and vasoconstrictive effects. See Table A.2 for infusion rates according to body weight	Preferable to give via a central line, since extravasation from a peripheral line may cause severe ischaemic injury due to vasoconstriction
Esmolol	As for atenolol	As for atenolol, plus: confusion, thrombophlebitis and skin necrosis from extravasation	Half-life = 9 min. Selective β_1-receptor antagonist. Onset of action occurs within 2 min. Following discontinuation, full recovery from beta-blockade effects occur at 18–30 min.	Give a loading dose of IV 500 µg/kg/min over 1 min before each titration step. Use titration steps of 50, 100, 150 and 200 µg/kg/min over 4 min each, stopping at the desired therapeutic effect	Can increase digoxin levels and prolong the action of suxamethonium. Interactions may occur with warfarin and intravenous morphine

			Metabolized by red blood cells		
Eptifibatide	Treatment of high-risk ACS	Bleeding and major bleeding Hypotension	Half-life = 150 min. Renal elimination	IV bolus 180 µg/kg followed by infusion at 2 µg/kg/min for up to 72h. Reduce dose if GFR < 50	Thrombocytopenia occurs in 0.2–1.2% of patients
Flecainide	Acute termination of atrial fibrillation Accessory pathway tachycardias	QRS prolongation, pro-arrhythmic, negatively inotropic, dizziness, visual disturbances, ataxia, peripheral neuropathy, reversible increase in liver enzymes	Half-life = 13–19h. Two-thirds hepatically metabolized, one-third excreted unchanged in the urine	IV 2 mg/kg or maximum 150mg over 10–30min. Maintenance infusion 1.5mg/kg/h (in 5% dextrose or normal saline) for 1h, subsequently reduced to 100–250 µg/kg/h for up to 24h. Maximum cumulative dose in first 24h = 600mg	Contraindications: sick sinus syndrome, left ventricular dysfunction, intraventricular conduction delay or AV block, patients with a history of ACS. Can increase stimulation threshold in patients with permanent pacemakers, therefore use with caution. If QRS complex is prolonged by 20% from baseline, reduce dose or discontinue, until ECG returns to normal
Fondaparinux	Medical treatment of ACS	Major and minor bleeding	Half-life = 17–21 hours. Peak activity after 2 h. Renal elimination	2.5 mg subcutaneously od for up to 8 days	Heparin should be given during PCI to prevent catheter-related thrombus

Appendix A: (Contd)

Drug	Indication	Side effects	Pharmacokinetics	Dosing regimen	Comments/Cautions/Contraindications
Glucagon	Reversal of beta-blockade side effects unresponsive to atropine	Nausea, vomiting, diarrhoea, hypokalaemia	Half-life = 5 min. Metabolized and cleared by the liver and kidney	50–150 µg/kg in 5% dextrose as an IV bolus over at least 1 min. If the response is not maintained, a further bolus dose may be required (or an infusion in 5% dextrose of 1–5 mg/h)	
Glyceryl trinitrate (GTN)	Treatment of angina. Left ventricular failure and pulmonary oedema. Hypertensive emergencies	Hypotension, headache, dizziness, flushing	Half-life = 1–4 min. Metabolized mainly by the liver and blood to dinitrates which are less potent	50 mg in 50 mL of solution as supplied by the manufacturer. Begin infusion at 10 µg/min (0.6 mL/h), increase by 10 µg/min every 15 min until a therapeutic effect is obtained. Maximum dose is 200 µg/min (12 mL/h)	Contraindications: hypotension, hypertropic obstructive cardiomyopathy, severe aortic or mitral stenosis, cardiac tamponade, constrictive pericarditis, cerebral haemorrhage. Tolerance with sustained blood levels
Insulin	Hyperglycaemia	Hypoglycaemia, hypokalaemia		50 U of short-acting insulin (i.e. Actrapid or Humulin S) in 50 mL normal saline. Administer according to sliding scale (see Table A.3)	

Drug	Indications	Adverse effects	Notes	Dose	Cautions
Isoprenaline	Heart block Severe bradycardia	Tachycardia, arrhythmias, hypotension, hypokalaemia, hyperglycaemia, headache, tremor, sweating	Half-life = 2 min. Adrenergic agonist $\beta_1 > \beta_2$	5 mg in 500 mL 5% dextrose or saline (concentration of 10 μg/mL), infuse at 0.5 mL/min (5 μg/min). Increase infusion rate to 1 mL/min to maintain adequate ventricular rate. The usual upper limit is 2 mL/min (20 μg/min). Isoprenaline is only used to maintain cardiac output until transvenous or transcutaneous pacing can be established	Caution: ischaemic heart disease, diabetes mellitus, and hyperthyroidism. Can increase infarct size and produce tachyarrhythmias
Isosorbide dinitrate	Angina Left ventricular failure	As for GTN	Half-life = 10 h. Metabolized by the liver to active mononitrate, excreted by the kidney	50 mg in 50 mL of solution as supplied by the manufacturer. Infuse between 2 and 10 mg/h. Maximum dose = 20 mg/h	As for GTN
Labetalol	Blood pressure control in hypertensive emergencies or acute aortic dissection	As for atenolol	Half-life = 3–4 h. High lipid solubility, not cardioselective, α-blockade effect, metabolized by the liver	50 mg slow IV bolus over 1 min, repeat after 5 min if necessary (maximum 200 mg). For continuous infusion, commence infusion rate at 15 mg/h and every 30–60 min up to 160 mg/h. Discontinue infusion once blood	As for atenolol

Appendix A: (Contd)

Drug	Indication	Side effects	Pharmacokinetics	Dosing regimen	Comments/Cautions/Contraindications
				pressure falls to desired level and initiate oral therapy	
Lignocaine (lidocaine)	Ventricular tachycardia Ventricular fibrillation	CNS side effects including dizziness, paraesthesiae, drowsiness, confusion, convulsions and respiratory depression, hypotension, bradycardia	Effect of a single bolus lasts only a few minutes, then half-life = 2 h. Rapid hepatic metabolism	50 mg bolus over a few minutes. Can be repeated to a maximum of 200 mg. Follow up with an infusion of 4 mg/min for 30 min, then 2 mg/min for 2 h, then 1 mg/min over 24 h (500 mg in 500 mL 5% dextrose, gives a concentration of 1 mg/mL)	Reduce concentration in hepatic failure, congestive cardiac failure, following cardiac surgery and shock. Cimetidine and beta-blockers can increase blood levels
Magnesium sulphate	Persistent ventricular tachyarrhythmias Polymorphic ventricular tachycardia	Nausea, flushing, hypotension, confusion, weakness, loss of tendon reflexes, arrhythmias	Excreted by the kidney	Arrhythmias: 4 mL of 50% magnesium sulphate (8 mmol) in 100 mL of 5% dextrose or normal saline IV. Repeat once if necessary. MI*: 8 mmol bolus over 20 min, followed by an infusion of 65–72 mmol over 24 h	Caution in renal failure and liver problems *The evidence to support the routine administration of intravenous magnesium in acute MI is controversial, and therefore the use of magnesium should be restricted to the treatment of recurrent ventricular arrhythmias

Metoprolol	As for atenolol	As for atenolol	Half-life = 3–7 h. Partially lipid soluble, cardioselective, metabolized by the liver	IV 2.5 mg over 2–4 min. May repeat every 5 min up to 15 mg	As for atenolol
Naloxone	To reverse respiratory depression induced by opioids	Nausea, vomiting, sweating, tachycardias. Can precipitate an acute withdrawal syndrome and non-cardiogenic pulmonary oedema in addicts	Half-life = 60–90 min; therefore, short duration of action. Onset of action within 1–2 min following IV injection. Metabolized by the liver	Opioid overdose: 0.8–2 mg IV, repeated at intervals of 2–3 min to a maximum of 10 mg. For a continuous infusion: 2 mg diluted in 500 mL 5% dextrose or normal saline (4 μg/mL), start infusion at 60% of the initial administered dose per hour	The duration of action of all opioids is often greater than that of naloxone; therefore, additional doses (or a continuous IV infusion) of naloxone may be required. The patient should be closely observed following initial reversal Use with caution in patients with pre-existing cardiovascular disease or in patients receiving cardiotoxic drugs, since arrhythmias (VT, VF, atrial fibrillation) can occur
Noradrenaline (nor-epinephrine)	To improve blood pressure in hypotensive patients by causing peripheral vasoconstriction	Hypertension, headache, palpitations, bradycardia, arrhythmias, peripheral ischaemia,	Half-life = 3 min. Except in the heart, its action is predominantly on α-receptors	Comes as a strong sterile solution (2 mg/mL). Make up a concentration of 80 μg/mL by adding 4 mg (2 mL solution) to 48 mL of 5% dextrose, or 40 mg (20 mL solution) to 480 mL 5%	Contraindications: hypertension, pregnancy, patients on monoamine oxidase inhibitors. Caution in patients with ischaemic heart disease

Appendix A: (*Contd*)

Drug	Indication	Side effects	Pharmacokinetics	Dosing regimen	Comments/Cautions/ Contraindications
		extravasation can cause necrosis		dextrose (this gives a concentration of 80 μg/mL). Normal saline can also be used. The usual infusion dose ranges between 0.01 and 0.5 μg/kg/min. Higher infusion doses are acceptable depending on the clinical condition	
Potassium chloride	Hypokalaemia	Arrhythmias		Add 20–60 mmol/L to 100 mL or 250 mL 5% dextrose or normal saline. Infuse at a rate no greater than 30 mmol/h. Concentrated solutions may be irritant and painful, therefore administer centrally if possible	Contraindicated in renal failure
Propranolol	As for atenolol	As for atenolol	Half life = 1–6 h. Lipid soluble, non-cardioselective, metabolized by the liver	IV 0.5–1 mg every 5 min to a maximum of 0.15–0.2 mg/kg	As for atenolol

| Reteplase (Rapilysin, r-PA) | STEMI | Minor and major haemorrhages, and hypersensitivity reactions (allergic reactions) | Half-life = 15min. Recombinant plasminogen activator which catalyses the cleavage of endogenous plasminogen to generate plasmin. Primarily eliminated by the kidney and to a small extent by the liver; however, no dose change is required in renal or hepatic insufficiency | Reconstitute 10U in 10mL of the solvent provided (using the filter supplied). Give slowly over 2min. Administer a further 10U after 30min. Give heparin IV 5000U before commencing r-PA, followed by 1000U/h after completion of the second r-PA bolus dose. Aim for an aPTT 50–75s (1.5–2.5 times control) | At present, few absolute contraindications as many are now relative, which needs interpreting within the clinical context. See section on thrombolysis, in Chapter 1 |
| Sodium bicarbonate | Prolonged resuscitation (pH <7.1 or base excess $\leq$ −10) | Tissue necrosis if extravasated. Administration can result in the generation of carbon dioxide, which diffuses rapidly into cells. This can result in a paradoxical intracellular acidosis; a negative inotropic effect on ischaemic myocardium; a high, osmotically active, | | 50mL of 8.4% (50 mmol/L) by slow intravenous injection | Do not administer via an endotracheal tube. Avoid adding to solutions containing calcium chloride or calcium gluconate. Use separate IV access |

Appendix A: (*Contd*)

Drug	Indication	Side effects	Pharmacokinetics	Dosing regimen	Comments/Cautions/Contraindications
		sodium load to an already compromised circulation and brain; and a left shift in the oxygen dissociation curve, inhibiting release of oxygen to the tissues			
Sodium nitroprusside	Hypertensive crisis	Hypotension, cyanide or cyanate accumulation, lactic acidosis, hypoxia, headache, dizziness, abdominal pain, perspiration, palpitations, phlebitis	Rapid action, pre- and after load reduction. Effects wear off 1–10 min after discontinuation. Metabolized to thiocyanate and excreted by the kidney (2.7–7 days). Degraded by light	Add 50 mg to 500 mL of 5% dextrose (concentration 100 µg/mL). Prepare solution immediately prior to use, and protect from light during administration. Initial dose (in a patient not already taking antihypertensive treatment): 0.3 µg/kg/min adjusting by increments of 0.5 µg/kg/min every 5 min to a range between 0.5 and 8 µg/kg/min. Maintain a blood pressure at 30–40%	Caution in hypothyroidism, renal impairment, hyponatraemia, IHD, impaired cerebral circulation. Contraindications: severe hepatic impairment, severe vitamin B12 deficiency. If infused for >24 h, give vitamin B12 (hydroxycobalamin, 1 mg, IM). Check serum thiocyanate concentration (toxic level >100 µg/mL) or monitor blood gases for metabolic acidosis

Drug	Indication	Pharmacology	Adverse effects	Dose	Notes
				lower than pre-treatment diastolic BP. Fresh solution is required every 4h, or earlier if it becomes discoloured. Duration of therapy should not exceed 72h, and sudden withdrawal should be avoided. Terminate infusion over 15–30 min	
Streptokinase	STEMI Pulmonary embolism (PE)	Half-life = 30 min. Activates plasminogen	Minor and major haemorrhages, hypotension, rash, nausea and vomiting, allergic reactions including anaphylaxis, fever	MI: 1.5 million units in 100mL normal saline over 1h PE: 250 000 units over 30min, then 100 000 units every hour for up to 12–72h. Monitor clotting parameters	At present, few absolute contraindications as many are now relative, which needs interpreting within the clinical context. See section on thrombolysis, in Chapter 1
Tenecteplase (TNKase, TNK-tpa)	STEMI	Half-life 20–24 min. Derivative of human tissue plasminogen activator that binds to fibrin and converts plasminogen to plasmin	Minor and major haemorrhages, and hypersensitivity reactions (allergic reactions)	Tenecteplase is dosed based on weight and is given as a single-bolus injection over 5 s (<60 kg = 30mg, 60–69 kg = 35 mg, 70–79 kg = 40mg, 80–89 kg = 45mg, 90 kg = 50mg). Tenecteplase is supplied as a sterile, lyophilized powder in a 50-mg vial. Each 50-mg vial of tenecteplase is packaged with one 10-mL vial of sterile water for injection,	This drug is not compatible with dextrose, and therefore should not be given in the same intravenous line. Lines containing dextrose should be flushed before and after administration. At present, few absolute contraindications as many are now relative, which needs interpreting within the clinical context. See

Appendix A: (*Contd*)

Drug	Indication	Side effects	Pharmacokinetics	Dosing regimen	Comments/Cautions/Contraindications
				for reconstitution. Give heparin bolus of 4000 U and infusion of 800 U/h for patients <67 kg; 5000 U bolus and infusion of 1000 U/h for patients >67 kg. Continue infusion for at least 48 h. Aim for an aPTT: 50–75 s (1.5–2.5 times control)	section on thrombolysis, in Chapter 1
Tirofiban	High-risk ACS	Major and minor bleeding. Thrombocytopenia	Half-life = 1.8 h. Renal excretion	IV infusion of 0.4 μg/kg/min for 30 min followed by infusion of 0.1 μg/kg/min for 48 h. High-dose bolus tirofiban is an IV bolus of 25 μg/kg/min over 3 min followed by 0.15 μg/kg/min for 18 h. Half infusion dose if GFR < 30	Incidence of thrombocytopenia 0.4–1.9%
Verapamil	Narrow complex tachycardia (SVT) where adenosine is contraindicated or has failed	Sinus or AV nodal inhibition. Negatively inotropic	Half-life = 4–6 h. Liver metabolized. Active metabolite norverapamil	5–10 mg over 2 min. A further 5 mg can be given after 5–10 min	Contraindications: hypotension, bradycardia, second and third degree AV block, sick sinus syndrome, cardiogenic shock, cardiac failure, broad complex tachycardia

Explanation of abbreviations can be found in the abbreviations list on pages vii–viii.

Table A.1 Dobutamine administration. Add 250 mg (5 mL of 50 mg/mL solution) in 45 mL of 5% dextrose or normal saline (giving a concentration of 5000 μg/mL). Commence infusion at 2.5 μg/kg/min initially, slowly increasing to a maximum of 20 μg/min. The following table gives infusion rates in mL/h for a solution of 5000 μg/mL according to dose required and body weight

Dobutamine infusion rate (μg/kg/min)	Body weight (kg)				
	50	60	70	80	90
2.5	1.5	1.8	2.1	2.4	2.7
5	3.0	3.6	4.2	4.8	5.4
10	6.0	7.2	8.4	9.6	10.8
15	9.0	10.8	12.6	15.4	16.2
20	12	14.4	16.8	19.2	21.6

Table A.2 Dopamine administration. Add 400 mg (10 mL of 40 mg/mL solution) to 40 mL of 5% dextrose to give a total volume of 50 mL, and a drug concentration of 8000 μg/mL. The following table gives infusion rates in mL/h for an 8000 μg/mL solution according to dose required and body weight

Dopamine infusion rate (μg/kg/min)	Body weight (kg)				
	50	60	70	80	90
2.5	0.9	1.1	1.3	1.5	1.7
5	1.9	2.3	2.6	3.0	3.4
10	3.8	4.5	5.2	6.0	6.8
15	5.7	6.8	7.8	9.0	10.2
20	7.6	9.0	10.4	12.0	13.6

Table A.3 Short-acting insulin (Actrapid) sliding scale. Add 50 units of Actrapid in 50 mL of normal saline to give a concentration of 1 unit/mL. The following table gives the infusion rates depending on the BMs

BM stick	Insulin infusion rate (units/h)
<5	0[a]
5.1–10	1
10.1–15	2
15.1–20	3
>20	6 (and urgent diabetologist review)

[a]Insulin-dependent diabetics require a maintenance infusion of 0.5 units/h.

APPENDIX B: LABORATORY VALUES AND USEFUL FORMULAE

Laboratory values	
Biochemistry	**Reference range**
Na	135–145 mmol/L
K	3.5–5 mmol/L
Cl	95–105 mmol/L
Mg	0.75–1.05 mmol/L
Urea	2.5–6.5 mmol/L
Creatinine	70–120 mmol/L
Creatinine clearance	80–140 mL/min
Bicarbonate	24–30 mmol/L
Fasting glucose	3.5–5.5 mmol/L
Calcium (total)	2.12–2.65 mmol/L
Calcium (ionized)	1.0–1.25 mmol/L
Phosphate	0.8–1.45 mmol/L
Alanine aminotransferase	5–35 iu/L
Alkaline phosphatase	30–300 iu/L (adults)
Bilirubin	3–17 μmol/L
Albumin	35–50 g/L
Aspartate transaminase (AST)	5–35 iu/L
Lactic dehydrogenase (LDH)	70–250 iu/L
Creatine kinase (CK)[a]	25–195 iu/L (males) 25–170 iu/L (females)
CK-MB mass	<5 μg/L
CK-MB mass:CK ratio	>3 (MI likely)
Troponin T	<0.05 μg/L
Troponin I[b]	<0.1 μg/L
C reactive protein	<8 mg/L

Continued

Free T4	9–22 pmol/L
TSH	0.5–5.7 mu/L

[a]CK values in healthy Afro-Caribbeans may be increased 2–3 times the quoted reference limit.
[b]Assay dependent, therefore check reference in laboratory.

Arterial blood gases	Reference range
pH	7.35–7.44
PaO_2	12–14.7 kPa[a]
$PaCO_2$	4.7–6.0 kPa[a]
HCO_3	23–33 mmol/L
O_2 saturation	93–98%
H[1]	36–44 mmol/L
Base excess	±2 mmol/L

[a]7.6 mmHg = 1 kPa.

Haematology	Reference range
Hb	13.5–18.0 g/dL (males)
	11.5–16.0 g/dL (females)
WCC	4–11 3 10^9/L
Neutrophils	2–7.5 3 10^9/L
	40–75% WCC
Lymphocytes	1.3–3.5 3 10^9/L
	20–45% WCC
Eosinophils	0.04–0.44 3 10^9/L
	1–6% WCC
Basophils	0–0.1 3 10^9/L
	0–1% WCC
ESR (increases with age)	<20 mm in 1 hour (rough guide) Age ÷ 2 (males) (Age + 10) ÷ 2 (females)

Platelets	$150–400 \times 10^9/L$
Prothrombin time	10–14 s
aPTT	35–45 s
Fibrinogen	2–4.5 g/L
FDPs	<10 mg/L

Haemodynamic pressures and parameters	Reference range
Left ventricle	
Systolic	100–140 mmHg
End diastolic	3–12 mmHg
Right ventricle	
Systolic	15–30 mmHg
End diastolic	2–8 mmHg
Aortic	
Systolic	100–140 mmHg
Diastolic	60–90 mmHg
Mean (diastolic + 1/3 pulse pressure)[a]	70–105 mmHg
Pulmonary artery	
Systolic	15–30 mmHg
Diastolic	4–12 mmHg
Mean	9–18 mmHg
Wedge (left atrium)	
Mean	2–12 mmHg
A wave	3–15 mmHg
V wave	2–10 mmHg
Right atrium	
Mean	2–8 mmHg
A wave	2–10 mmHg

V wave	2–10 mmHg
Systemic vascular resistance	700–1600 dyn $\times$ s $\times$ cm^{-5}
Total pulmonary resistance	100–300 dyn $\times$ s $\times$ cm^{-5}
Pulmonary vascular resistance	20–130 dyn $\times$ s $\times$ cm^{-5}
Cardiac output	5.5–9 L/min
Cardiac index	2.6–4.2 L/min/m^2

[a]Pulse pressure = difference between systolic and diastolic pressures.

Electrocardiography and echocardiography	Reference range
P wave width	<110 ms (lead II)
P wave height	<2.5 mm (lead II)
PR interval	120–200 ms
QRS duration	<120 ms
QT interval[a]	440 ms (males) 460 ms (female)
Aortic root	2–3.7 cm
Aortic cusp separation	1.5–2.6 cm
Left atrium	1.9–4 cm
Left ventricle diameter (end systole)	2.5–4.1 cm
Left ventricle diameter (end diastole)	3.5–5.6 cm
Left ventricular posterior wall thickness (end systole)	0.9–1.3 cm
Left ventricular posterior wall thickness (end diastole)	0.7–1.1 cm
Interventricular septal wall thickness (end systole)	0.9–1.8
Interventricular septal wall thickness (end diastole)	0.7–1.1 cm
Right ventricle (end diastole)	2.3 cm
Ratio of septum to posterior wall thickness	1.3:1
Fractional shortening	30–40%
Ejection fraction	50–85%

[a]When using drugs known to prolong the QT interval, discontinue or reduce dose if QT interval is greater than 500 ms or increases by more than 60 ms from baseline.

Formulae

Bazett's formula (corrected QT interval)	$= \dfrac{\text{QT interval (seconds)}}{\text{RR internal (seconds)}}$
LDL-cholesterol (Friedwald's equation)	$= \text{Total cholesterol} - \dfrac{\text{(triglyceride 1 HDL - cholesterol)}}{2.19}$

(Formula only valid for triglyceride concentrations < 4.5 mmol/L)

Cockroft and Gault formula for estimating
creatinine clearance (mL/min) =

$$\frac{(140 - \text{age in years}) \times (\text{weight in kg})}{72 \times \text{serum creatinine in mg / dL}}$$

(for women multiply formula by 0.85; mg/dL = μmol/L $\div$ 88.4)

$$\text{Body surface area} = \sqrt{\frac{\text{Height (cm)} \times \text{Weight (kg)}}{3600}}$$

APPENDIX C: USEFUL WEB ADDRESSES

General	URL address	Content
American College of Cardiology	http://www.acc.org/	Clinical statements, ACC/AHA practice guidelines, links to other online cardiology journals, ECG of the month, echo of the month
BNF	http://www.bnf.org/	Drugs in the British National Formulary
British Cardiac Society	http://www.bcs.com/	BCS guidelines, meetings, education and training issues
Cardiac angiograms and coronary arteriograms	http://www.sbu.ac.uk/dirt/museum/gs-sixth.html#11	Developed by South Bank University and contains normal and abnormal cardiac angiograms
Cardiac arrhythmias	http://www.arrhythmia.net/	Case histories, ECGs, diagnosis and management of various cardiac arrhythmias
Cardiology Compass	http://www.cardiologycompass.com/	A general overview of various cardiology procedures, image bank, links to other online cardiology journals and resources
Cardiosource	http://www.cardiosource.com/	Cardiology information resource service for cardiovascular news, clinical trials, Medline, trial acronyms, journal links (including the American College of Cardiology journal and Current Journal Review Scan), ACC/AHA practice guidelines
Doctors.net.uk	http://www.doctors.net.uk/	General medical information including cardiology forum, presentations, access to *Clinical Medicine* by P Kumar and M Clark, *Clinical Biochemistry* by William Marshall, *Textbook of Paediatrics* by Forfar and Arneil, *Merck Manual of Diagnosis and Therapy*, NICE and SIGN guidelines, Clinical Risk Management, TRIP, *Hospital Medicine* journal and many more useful links
Doctorsworld.com	http://www.doctorsworld.com	General medical news, career information, a library which includes access to guidelines, formularies, clinical calculators, Merck's manual, *Gray's Anatomy*, *Emergency Medicine*, *Travel Medicine* and many more

ECG library	http://www.mrcppart1.co.uk/ecgs/ecghome.html	Excellent collection of ECGs
Electronic Medicines Compendium	http://emc.vhn.net	Provides free access to up-to-date, comprehensive and reliable information about prescription and over-the-counter medicines available in the UK
Emergency Medicine on the Web	http://www.ncemi.org/	Extensive resource on the management of acute medical emergencies. From e-medicine online textbooks, algorithms, calculators, nomograms, scoring systems, tables, key journals update, online dictionaries and many other useful links
European Society of Cardiology	http://www.escardio.org/	Educational resources, clinical statements, ESC guidelines
Freemedicaljournals.com	http://www.freemedicaljournals.com/	Access to available free online journals
Freewarepalm.com	http://freewarepalm.com/medical/medical.shtml	A collection of medical programmes such as drug databases, calculators, eponyms, biochemistry and haematology interpretation assistance, etc., that can be downloaded and used in a handheld computer
InCirculation.net	http://www.incirculation.net/frame.asp	Cardiology information resource service. Up to date reports on publications of interest, image bank, links to other useful websites and online journals
Lipidhealth	http://www.lipidhealth.org/	Issues regarding lipid management
Medicdirect.co.uk	http://www.dr.medicdirect.co.uk/main.ihtml	General medical resource centre. Lectures, slide library, leading edge articles, prescribers' journal online, drug update, career advice, clinical guidelines, clinical tools, clinical calculators and scores, patient information and videos
Medicines and Drug Information Centre	http://www.digri.demon.co.uk/drugs.htm	Excellent collection of links on drug information, from general prescribing to individual properties, adverse reactions and interactions

Appendix C: (Contd)

General	URL address	Content
Medscape.com	http://www.medscape.com/	General medical resource service with the option of receiving updates in chosen specialty
National library of medicine	http://www.nlm.nih.gov/	Medline, PubMed, Medline plus
North American Society for Pacing and Electrophysiology (NASPE)	http://www.naspe.org/	Heart rhythm information and resource for healthcare professionals and the public
QT Drugs.org	http://georgetowncert.org/qtdrugs.html	Drugs that prolong the QT interval
Resuscitation Council UK	http://www.resus.org.uk	A valuable resource for providing information on resuscitation, which is updated regularly. All new publications by the council are posted on the site together with details about forthcoming events, courses, membership and, when appropriate, important statements
The Cochrane Library	http://www.update-software.com/cochrane/cochrane-frame.html	Abstracts of Cochrane Reviews
The X-ray files	http://www.radiology.co.uk/xrayfile/xray/index.htm	A large collection of radiology cases, tutorials and useful links
Theheart.org	http://www.theheart.org/index.cfm	Cardiology information resource service. Up to date reports on publications of interest, image bank, links to other useful websites and online journals
Toxbase	http://www.spib.axl.co.uk/	Management of drug overdoses

Journals	URL address
Annals of Internal Medicine	http://www.annals.org/
British Medical Journal	http://www.bmj.com/
Chest	http://www.chestjournal.org/
Circulation	http://circ.ahajournals.org/
Clinical Cardiology	http://clinicalcardiology.org/
European Heart Journal	http://www.harcourt-international.com/journals/euhj/
Heart	http://heart.bmjjournals.com/
Hypertension	http://hyper.ahajournals.org/
Journal of Interesting EKGs	http://www.ekgreading.com/journal.htm
Journal of the American College of Cardiology	http://www.acc.org/
Journal of the American Medical Association	http://jama.ama-assn.org/
Lancet	http://www.thelancet.com/
New England Journal of Medicine	http://www.nejm.org/content/index.asp

INDEX

Page numbers in **bold type** refer to tables and boxes; those in *italic* to figures.